Older Workers in Europe

Older Workers in Europe

Edited by
Anthony Chiva and Jill Manthorpe

Open University Press

Open University Press
McGraw-Hill Education
McGraw-Hill House
Shoppenhangers Road
Maidenhead
Berkshire
England
SL6 2QL

email: enquiries@openup.co.uk
world wide web: www.openup.co.uk

and Two Penn Plaza, New York, NY 10121—2289, USA

first published 2009

A catalogue record of this book is available from the British Library

ISBN-13: 978 0 335 22275 9 (pb) 978 0 335 22276 6 (hb)
ISBN-10: 0 335 22275 7 (pb) 0 335 22276 5 (hb)

Typeset by Kerrypress Ltd, Luton, Bedfordshire
Printed and bound in the UK by Bell & Bain Ltd, Glasgow

The McGraw·Hill Companies

Contents

This book is dedicated to the many older people who have informed our understanding of later life. Also to David Stears who made an imaginative and dedicated commitment to health promotion and public health, and a good friend.

Figures

Tables

Contributors

Jo Aspland is a Research Assistant in the Faculty of Health and Social Care at the University of Hull. She has worked on a number of research projects focusing on equality and diversity. She has a first degree in Economics, an MSc in Engineering and a postgraduate certificate in Social Science Research Methods.

Anthony Chiva has worked in the education field for most of his career. This has been in the public and voluntary sectors, including schools, colleges, universities and the health service. Currently, he is working as Head of Education at Life Academy, formerly the Pre-Retirement Association. He has published in several key areas related to his interests in personal and spiritual development; specifically, skills management, health promotion, life planning and older workers.

Inés Domínguez López has been working for CREA (Aragon Business Employers Confederation), which is a Euro Info Centre in Zaragoza. She manages a number of European Projects, such as 50+ Europe and the EU Equal Project Promising Practices on reconciling family and professional life.

Elizabeth Farmer is a Chartered MCIPD and a Director of positivexperience Ltd. She was Director of Experience Works! (2002–2004), funded by the East Midlands Development Agency. Elizabeth was responsible for raising awareness in the region of the implications of an ageing workforce and encouraging employers to recruit older workers. She managed the regional rollout of Experience Works! She developed a positive approach and process to train older workers in the skills, knowledge and confidence necessary for them to get the work they wanted.

Matt Flynn is a Senior Lecturer at Middlesex University Business School in the UK. He has carried out research for the UK government, CIPD, TUC and ESRC on age discrimination and retirement. He has also participated in an EU-funded project on age, knowledge management and diversity. He is currently conducting two pieces of comparative research: one looking at age management in the UK and Germany, and the other comparing the experience of UK and Japanese older workers.

Philippe Gabriel was the National Coordinator for the 50+ Europe Leonardo Project, Director of the Centre Universitaire de Formation des Enseignants et des Formateurs (CUFEF, eng. University Training Center for Teachers and Trainers) Université d'Avignon et des Pays du Vaucluse, Teacher – Researcher/ Lecturer. His research interests are: assessment within existing educational systems and international comparison; Culture numérique Digital Culture; and Enseignement supérieur et Formation des enseignants/Higher Education and Teacher Education.

Helen Gibson is a Research Assistant in the Faculty of Health and Social Care at the University of Hull. She has experience of undertaking both qualitative and quantitative research, and has most recently contributed to projects looking at Black and Minority Ethnic Students, the Children and Young People's Voluntary and Community Sector and the Disability Rights Commission formal investigation into fitness standards in Nursing, Teaching and Social Work.

Patrick Grattan was formerly the Chief Executive of The Age and Employment Network (TAEN). Patrick founded TAEN in 1997 and was Chief Executive for 10 years to 2007. In 2002 he set up the Equality and Diversity Forum. He has had an influential role in policy on age, employment and training, and in the creation of the Equality and Human Rights Commission. Patrick has worked in the Diplomatic Service and Civil Service and in the oil industry, working in the UK, the USA and France.

Sarah Harper is Professor at the Institute of Ageing, University of Oxford. Her research covers the social implications of demographic ageing with particular emphasis on ageing workforces, late life work and retirement; migration and intergenerational relationships; and the multigenerational family. She is lead investigator for the Ageing Workforce Programme, and has recently completed a study on Extending Late Life Work exploring the transitions to self-employment of men and women in their 50s within the IT industry; Impact of Migration on Families programme which examines the impact of migrant female care labour on family structures and networks; and Family and Intergenerational Relationships Programme.

Grzegorz Karpiuk, MA is currently a university teacher at the University of Information Technology and Management in Rzeszow, Poland, specializing in project management and international trade relations. His professional experience in management and implementation of projects are funded by a range of European programmes, including Equal, Structural Funds, PHARE, Leonardo da Vinci and Socrates. The topics covered by the projects implemented include employment and social policy, human resource management, customization of training to unemployed people and development of e-learning courses.

Jumbo Klercq is International Coordinator of Strategy and Innovation, Stavoor, Driebergen (NL). He is currently coordinating on the PEFETE network

(Grundtvig 4) on senior citizens' education, the IMWI project (Grundtvig 1) on intercultural learning, the LACE project (Grundtvig 1) on active citizenship and the IPM project (Leonardo da Vinci pilot) on intergenerational portfolio management. He is a member of the executive board of EAEA 2002 and for the has been, last two years as Vice-President.

Asmund Lunde has been Director of the Centre for Senior Policy (CSP) since 1988. The CSP changed focus in 1991/2 from Preparation for Retirement to Age Management or Age Related HRM (in Norway often named Senior Policy). CSP seeks to improve older workers' status and increase possibilities in their working life. He has also been engaged in several EU projects.

Jill Manthorpe is Professor of Social Work and Director of the Social Care Workforce Research Unit, King's College London. She has wide experience of work with older people, researching into areas such as adult safeguarding, social care and dementia. She has published, edited and co-authored numerous texts on social work and mental health, and workforce interests include older workers, international mobility and discrimination.

Stephen McNair is Director of the Centre for Research into the Older Workforce. He is currently a member of the Surrey Local Learning and Skills Council. In the past he has chaired the Strategic Policy Committee of the Universities Association for Adult Continuing Education, and has been a member of the Workforce Skills Committee of the South East England Development Agency, the Cabinet Office's Academic Advisory Committee on the National Skills Strategy, the Widening Participation Committee of the Higher Education Funding Council, the National Advisory Group on Continuing Education and Lifelong Learning, and the National Guidance Council. He has worked as a consultant for the OECD, University for Industry and the BBC. His research interests include the older workforce and the relationship between learning and work.

Jo Moriarty is a Research Fellow and Deputy Director of the Social Care Workforce Research Unit, King's College London where she carries out a range of research into social work education and the social care workforce. Her recent work includes membership of the research team involved in the evaluation of the social work degree qualification in England and work for the General Social Care Council looking at progression rates among social work students. She has a long-standing interest in services for people with dementia and their carers, and in ethnicity and ageing.

Yvan Paris was a research assistant at the 50+ Europe Leonardo Project at the Centre Universitaire de Formation des Enseignants et des Formateurs (CUFEF, eng. University Training Center for Teachers and Trainers) Université d'Avignon et des Pays du Vaucluse, careers adviser and teacher. His research interest is in lifelong vocational guidance and teaching activity.

Chris Phillipson is Vice-Chancellor for Learning and Academic Development and Professor of Applied Social Studies and Social Gerontology, University of Keele. His current research interests include globalization and ageing, social exclusion and older people, and transitions from work to retirement. He is a past President of the British Society of Gerontology and a member of the Training and Development Board of the Economic and Social Research Council. He has been a visiting Professor to universities in Japan and the USA.

Adam Piekara, MA Eng. is Coordinator of the Technology Transfer Centre in Rzeszow and university teacher at the University of Information Technology and Management in Rzeszow, Poland. His professional experience is in business consulting, financial management, institutional capacity building and project and quality management. He was formerly a Director of the Business Support Centre in Rzeszow. He has wide expertise in European funds (ESF, PHARE and Leonardo da Vinci) and employment policy and is an Evaluator and Assessor of projects co-financed by the European funds.

Kerry Platman is a Senior Research Fellow at the Warwick Institute for Employment Research, University of Warwick. She specializes in the ageing of the workforce and its impact on employment and retirement practices. Her current research examines management practices and career transitions in the Information Technology sector. She speaks and writes about a range of issues associated with workforce ageing including the management of longer working lives; age discrimination in employment; the business impact of workforce ageing; flexible transitions into retirement; learning and training over the life course; age management and healthy working lives; and employment and care burdens in later life. She is currently part of three interdisciplinary research networks involving academic colleagues in the UK, Europe and North Amercia.

Jan Shepherd has extensive experience of teaching, training and staff development. When working at the University of Surrey, she coordinated the teacher training programme for the Post-16 Sector including training nurse tutors and lecturers. She has been actively involved and managed a wide range of European programmes. She was the European coordinator for a major Leonardo da Vinci project – 50+ Europe (www.50pluseurope.co.uk) which sought to overcome barriers to employment for the over 50s and for which the NHS was a key case study. This project contributed to the development of Intergenerational Portfolio Management project which she jointly coordinates in the UK for the Life Academy.

Jim Soulsby is Development Coordinator at the Association for Education and Ageing. Until recently he was Development Officer on the Older and Bolder Programme at NIACE. His research and development interests include Curriculum for Later Life, financial education for older people, employability in training for older people in the East Midlands region, age regulations and learning in care settings. He is also a Trustee for the Centre for Policy on Ageing (CPA) and Age Concern, Northamptonshire.

Anne Stimpson is a Research Associate in the Faculty of Health and Social Care at the University of Hull. She has a wide range of research experience utilizing qualitative and quantitative research methods. Her main research interests are care of older people including palliative care for the elderly and diabetes and dementia. She is particularly interested in the work-life experiences of older nurses and midwives and the reasons why they leave the professions.

Philip Taylor is Professor of Employment Policy in the Faculty of Business and Enterprise and Director of the Business, Work and Ageing Centre for Research at Swinburne University of Technology Australia. He was formerly a Senior Research Associate and Executive Director of Cambridge Interdisciplinary Research Centre on Ageing at the University of Cambridge. Philip is currently leading the BWA project 'Redesigning Work for an Ageing Society' which is supported by an ARC Linkages grant, the most substantial grant won to date by the Faculty of Business and Enterprise at Swinburne. His research interests are age and employment; individual orientations to work and retirement; employers' attitudes and practices towards older workers; and international developments in public policies aimed at combating age barriers in the labour market.

Jorge Alonso Vallejo has been working for CREA (Aragon Business Employers Confederation representing more than 26,000 SMEs) since 1994, as head of the International Department. He has managed several cooperation projects in Latin America, Asia and eastern Europe. He is a Member of the Enterprise Europe Network of the European Commission and holds an academic degree in Law and a master's degree in European Affairs. Previously he worked in the Spanish Employers Confederation in Brussels, Belgium. He has published books on 'European funding for the SMEs', 'the EU trademark', 'the EU and the Internal Market' and 'the enlarged EU'.

Roger Watson is Professor of Nursing, Centre for Health & Social Care Studies and Service Development, School of Nursing and Midwifery, University of Sheffield. Professor Watson is best known for the development of the Edinburgh Feeding Evaluation in Dementia scale which is now used in several countries, including the USA and Taiwan. His research interests are wide and he has also researched the areas of caring in nursing and work, and study-related stress in nurses and nursing students. He is well published in refereed journals and has published several textbooks on science in nursing, accountability and research methods. Since 2003 he has been Editor of the

Journal of Clinical Nursing (now Editor-in-Chief), currently rated fifth in the world of nursing journals. In 2007 he became the first UK nurse elected Fellow of the American Academy of Nursing.

Jane Wray is a Research Fellow in the Faculty of Health and Social Care at the University of Hull. Jane has undertaken research in the field of equality and diversity for the last 10 years. She works closely with organizations in the statutory and voluntary/community sector to promote inclusion of disabled people. She is particularly interested in access to the professions and fitness to practise and recently led a Disability Rights Commission-funded project examining decision-making on fitness standards in Nursing, Teaching and Social Work.

Acknowledgements

This book is the result of a collaboration between a wide range of professionals who work with many different and varied organizations. Our thanks go to these collaborative initiatives that underpin this text.

The editors would like to thank Joanna Walker and Rachel Gear for their support in developing this publication.

We would like to acknowledge the following sources of materials used in this edited collection: The Stationery Office and Office for National Statistics (ONS) survey and statistical data.

The research reported here would not have been possible without the funding received from a wide range of funding councils and charities, including the EU Leonardo da Vinci fund.

Foreword

Jumbo Klercq

Shifts and shadows of an ageing landscape

What is the meaning of a new book about *Older Workers in Europe*?

Currently, we are awaiting the final results of the large case study collection and analysis of employment initiatives for an ageing workforce in all 25 member states undertaken by the European Foundation for the Improvement of Living and Working Conditions. Sara E. Rix (2005) has already examined older worker employment and retirement trends in the European Union (EU) and in Japan. She concludes that the EU has set ambitious older worker employment goals for its member countries and has put pressure on these countries to reach the established targets.

The European Commission appealed in its Communication (EU 2004) 'Increasing the employment of older workers and delaying the exit from the labour market' to the member states to take *drastic action*. Not only 'a radical shift in policy measures, away from a culture of early retirement, towards comprehensive active ageing policies', but answering the challenge to enhance the employability of those currently in their 40s and 50s, as well at to ensure that greater numbers of those currently aged 55–64 stay in work.

This book reflects the paradigm shift in European and national policies focusing on the challenges for economy and world competitiveness caused by changing demographic profiles and an ageing workforce. The different chapters, written by excellent and deeply involved experts, explain to us the way these changes are getting more and more visible. The relevance of this book is that it shows us the first contours of a landscape in change, not only in terms of policy, but also in terms of practice.

We need to go back to 1996 when the first European project started, EuroWork Age, as a European network of agents to disseminate good practice concerning employment policy and the productive management of an ageing workforce (Delsen and Reday-Mulvey 1996). It was like looking for needles in a haystack, because the main practice over the last 20 years was exclusion of older workers from the labour market based on a simplistic and short-term policy, which resulted in the large-scale removal of 'older workers' via redundancy and early retirement in much of western Europe.

In 1998 the first National Action Plans on Employments were published and discussed in the European Council (EU Employment and Social Affairs 1998). The Commission also published its guidelines for the member states forcing them to include measures to retain and (re)integrate older workers in the labour market (EU 2005). This change from exclusion to inclusion is reflected in the 'flexibility agenda' which has permeated much of the current debate among policy-makers, opinion-formers and business leaders in the UK and in many other European countries.

The first part of this book explains the background and shows its evidence; the second part guides us into the current employment and labour market policies for an ageing workforce, and into initiatives in the workplace.

The third part of the book goes beyond policy and research and focuses on innovative practice. What is really changing? How does it function? What are the first results? What could be identified as success factors? What are the risks? Are initiatives in the workplace reflecting the changing minds of policy-makers? And what are the attitudes of older workers themselves? Older workers seem to be more positive about work and extending working life than is commonly assumed, but there are major differences in the workforce and the line-management is often much younger and not always capable and sensitive to identify older worker's needs.

This book shows us the way in which different actors in the UK have taken steps to make the labour market work better for those in their 40s, 50s and 60s. It points out that in other European countries also (50+ Europe 2004) a range of key actors needs to be involved in changing the patterns: employers, managers, human resource personnel, employment agencies and agents relating to employers; for example, professional bodies, social partners and Chambers of Commerce. Problems of an ageing workforce can only be solved in practice by social partners and supported by professional experts; changing policy can only facilitate innovation. Solutions can be found in local projects like 'Experience Works!' in East Midlands or in a sectoral approach like the lived experience of nurses and midwives in the NHS.

The third part of the book shows not only the success of innovation but also the paradoxes and the 'stubbornness' of practice. When we examine the new ageing landscape of the labour market, we see the change in patterns, and the new innovative initiatives, but we are discovering also new areas and issues. What will be the future options for older workers? Men and women leaving full-time employment in their 50s to take up self-employment, part-time and flexible working practices? Or people remaining within the full-time waged labour force, but facing a variety of pressures such as recruitment, retention and retraining through their own choice or through compulsory redundancy and/or involuntary early retirement?

When we are coming to these conclusions, we realize that it is time for critical reflection. Times are changing, policy is changing and this all creates its own dynamics. The economy itself is driving us forward. There is a new generation of older workers with other ambitions, other aspirations and other needs, more empowered and focused on their well-being. The political message of social inclusion is not always positive and implies new pressures and further key questions: What will be the benefits for older workers in this new landscape and how can they influence their own circumstances?

1 Introduction

Jill Manthorpe and Anthony Chiva

Older workers are the subject of this book and possibly the readership. Many of the contributors to this book also fall into the category of older worker. This is an unusual combination since policy and research, as well as human resources activity, often focus on problems, especially those belonging to other people. If we are to understand older workers, we need to understand ourselves and our own relationships with work.

It is well known, but only in some circles, that the drivers for the changes affecting older workers arise from demography (longevity, age cohort effects, fertility), globalization, economic pressures on social funds, the decreasing value of many pensions, legislative changes and the trends towards individual responsibility. To this should be added changes in the nature of work, attitudes to work and work patterns. The contributors to this book have been asked to reflect on these broadly but also to 'think out loud' about what these changes mean to particular places or work settings or to particular groups of people. We have also asked them to think beyond the UK to explore European factors if relevant. This is because the UK increasingly operates in a European context and the Europe workforce is more mobile, even in later life.

Governments across Europe have introduced major legislation concerning state retirement ages and pensions, but also incentive schemes for the retention and recruitment of older workers. In Chapter 9 Anthony Chiva and colleagues from across Europe outline some of these inducements. These changes in legislation have been strongly encouraged by the European Union (EU) so much so that each European member state has adopted age legislation since 2006. Changes in pension law are more complex across Europe, because of different ways that pensions are funded. In the UK recent changes in pension legislation enable workers to draw down their occupational pension, while also continuing in paid employment, even with the same employer. Is this the best model? Who benefits from this and why?

The demographic transition as populations age in many European countries (see Chapter 4) is more complex than originally envisaged. The trend to low birth rates continues despite flurries of interest around pronatalist policies. What is common to Old Europe is the important contribution younger migrants are making to their economies, with current large if selective migratory trends from eastern into western Europe. Many of these younger migrants are well qualified and some of the anticipated skills gaps and labour shortages have been reduced by this transnational movement of labour. But are such migrants transitory and affected more by currency fluctuations than labour market conditions? Are they concentrated in work where there are skills shortages? And will they themselves become older workers in the areas where they have moved to or will they return to their areas of origin? Migratory patterns are complex and unpredictable when just thinking of migrants within the EU. They become even more difficult to plan for when we include economic migrants from other areas of the world and refugees from many different continents who participate in the world of work in officially recognized but also unrecognized positions in the submerged economy.

These collective trends and counter trends are leading to a period of discouraged retirement (Phillipson et al. 2004) with governments and some employers across western Europe seeking to delay retirement as a way of managing their economies and social structures. Some key questions covered by contributors to this book include:

- How do older workers envisage their own lives?
- How does the challenge to early retirement play out?
- What economic drivers affect individuals' decisions to retire or work?
- What impacts will there be on social or human capital, such as volunteering or caring?
- How will employers react to requests to remain in the workforce from people reaching 65 years?
- What are the implications for training or retraining of older workers?
- How will the many trends of work and retirement impact on retention?

This book provides partial answers to many of these questions, drawing on state-of-the-art knowledge but also from ideas about work practices. In this introductory chapter, we provide an overview and context into which each chapter adds insight and depth. It may also trigger readers' own thinking and hopefully provide insights for employment practice in this field.

Identity

The challenges to older workers themselves at this time are significant and operate across many life dimensions. One such challenge is to the social identity of the older worker at this time of changing roles, role confusion and possible rolelessness. Chris Phillipson in Chapter 8 describes this as a period of transition and a subjective state of possible ambiguity. For some people their retirement plans may falter or fail but workplaces vary in their willingness to maintain continued employment. For others this period may be a time when they are valued in the labour market and yet face possibly welcome pulls from other areas of life: to become more actively (re)engaged with their families or social networks; to take up opportunities for new experiences, such as travel while they can; or to build up a second or third career or set of skills. Not everyone will want to be an older worker and other aspects of their social identity may be more valued. Will Chris Phillipson's calls for a redefinition of midlife be heeded? We are hopeful, as terms such as midlife and even later life are often far too vague and possibly pessimistic.

Rights to work

Current UK legislation on age does not require an employer to provide a justification for not employing a person aged over 65. This potentially weakens the position of an employee wishing to remain in work post-65. It will be interesting to observe case law as it emerges. In Chapter 4 Philip Taylor explores experiences from other countries that have already addressed some of these trends. Lessons from other countries are valuable in charting whose rights are recognized and of course, in Europe, many companies have multinational interests and may seek uniformity of working cultures. Likewise, professional bodies and trade unions talk to each other. Will these be the forums for older workers to share experiences and develop bargaining strategies? This may be a means to balance one of the risks that Philip Taylor foresees, that older people are treated as a reserve army of labour with minimal rights and low expectations about their abilities to shape the work they are called on to do. As he observes, there may be a need for older workers to move from being less passive in terms of the work and opportunities they are 'given' and become more active in negotiating what they can contribute and how.

The question of rights to work in later life begins to change conceptualizations of matters that often have been seen by employers as retention questions. While the factors affecting retention of labour, skills and human capital vary from sector to sector, with specific skills gaps and labour shortages, and sometimes excesses or abundance of some skills and personnel, retention is multifaceted. Older workers are sometimes able to negotiate their terms and actively choose to retain their links with their employer. Rights to work that is flexible, part time or selective have long been available to some professionals and may be ways in which older workers more generally seek to balance work-life demands and priorities. Generations that are familiar with maternity and latterly paternity rights may seek to build on such expectations.

The desire of people to continue working after 65 is neither uniform nor stable among individuals or across all sectors. In Chapter 3 Matt Flynn and Stephen McNair point to differing desires and values. Large-scale surveys are hugely informative and we hope for more longitudinal studies to see if or how views change over time, with accompanying explanatory models about what works and for whom.

Workplace influences

Older workers of course are but one side of the coin and some key questions need to be considered about retention practices and the creation of unemployed older people who may feel unemployable. Kerry Platman, in Chapter 5, reminds us of the importance of technological industries and enterprises in Europe, and ways in which young industries may privilege youth and its attributes. A knowledge economy is greatly prized but it may associate knowledge with innovation, and older workers with conservatism and redundancy. And in some definitions of older workers, the age may be lower than many of us would expect. Age groups are important but do not necessarily mean the same thing when talking about older workers and Chapter 10 reveals that while many European governments have stated policies about the retention of older people and their encouragement back to the workforce, they are applying these to different age cohorts.

Which employers and in which sectors will seek to retain older employees? Possibly not those areas where there has been great shedding of labour, but if regeneration is primed then labour markets may need filling. The example of the East Midlands region of England is one illustration of this and, in Chapter 10, Elizabeth Farmer and Jim Soulsby outline how local regional agencies sought to work together to equip older people to re-enter the workforce. This chapter further provides discussion of activities at a regional level which are important across Europe where regional governance and investment can be sizeable.

Feminization

The picture of recruitment and retraining of older workers is evolving in different sectors and industries. Health services have taken a lead in this area; not for altruistic reasons necessarily but because they face tremendous labour shortages. The working experiences of older nurses and midwives in the NHS are the focus of Chapter 11. Here Jo Aspland and her colleagues provide insight into strategies being adopted by health services faced by a combination of ageing workforces and steady demands for health care from ageing populations. In Chapter 6, older workers in social care services are considered for the first time in detail to the best of our knowledge. Jill Manthorpe and Jo Moriarty note that this sector is expanding and many vacancies in western Europe are currently being filled by migrant workers, with little attention to the potential of older workers. This is an area that may change considerably in some states. For example, in the UK, many local government-employed social care workers, in the main women, have been moved into the commercial sector of care where pensionable work is uncommon. The legacy of this for their retirement is concerning. Likewise, in many EU states, greater numbers of older people and their families are employing their own social care workers to help with day-to-day support. What will be the impact of this on older female workers? Will they greet such moves as providing flexible and rewarding work or will they regret the passing of teamwork and feel that they may be exploited by working in areas where hard won gains of health and safety may be less enforceable?

As both chapters on health care and social care make clear, these areas contain major employers and their employees are often women. Studies of older workers in Europe or elsewhere do not often focus on gender, despite the workforce profiles. In both health and social care, this elides over the gendered nature of work, where low wages accompany quite high skill levels and part-time work is not necessarily associated with low skills. Even when skills are in short supply, wages do not necessarily rise, and resources for later life may be limited. The general trend of solo living in later life in many European countries, through increased divorce and partnership breakdown, means that older women are often at risk of poverty with all the social exclusions and health problems that this may entail.

Workplace health

Sarah Harper in Chapter 2 reminds us that differences between skilled and unskilled work continue to be associated, of course, with financial remuneration and control over work. The political economies of work and retirement changed over the twentieth and early twenty-first centuries, with ebbing and flowing patterns of encouraged and discouraged retirement. The concept of a 'dependency ratio' is used to 'worry' the unwary, and possibly to manipulate ideas about ageing and older people. The dependency ratio provides a very simple form of analysis that may be used for planning purposes. However, it ignores the less visible economic contributions of older workers to family, neighbourhoods and civic concerns. The discourses on productive ageing

(Meadows and Volterra Consulting 2004) are helpful in demonstrating the direct contributions that older workers make to workplaces and communities. Social capital is not necessarily confined to neighbourhoods and families but can operate widely.

As Patrick Grattan observes in Chapter 7, the role of work in promoting health is underdeveloped. It is increasingly accepted that work has a role in promoting good mental or physical health or wellness, though how this applies to older workers is not so clear. For policy-makers one key question is how to develop or sustain coping strategies among the coming generations of older people. Policy is often accused of being short term but health is one area where there is increasingly interest in forecasting and future proofing, with due acknowledgements of the limits of such approaches. Interventions may have a sound economic rationale, since good mental and physical health in later lives benefits everyone; it maximizes the contributions of society that older people can make and they bring benefits to society by reducing the costs of poor mental health in later life (Cuijpers et al. 2006: 16–17).

In policy terms support may be focused on particular groups of older people whose resilience or coping may have been compromised by limited investment in their well-being and the ill-effects, damage and distress of harsh work or unemployment. Loss of peer and social networks or diminishing ones after retirement or redundancy are not an area of public policy that has traditionally received more than token efforts. Policy commitment to tackling social isolation and loneliness in later life may need to be thought about in the context of what happens to people during the latter periods of their working lives. Not everyone has a family, and relationships in the neighbourhood may be hard to build up if working life is busy and hours of travel are long. As Phillipson et al. (2004) observe, government policy impacts on vulnerable older people in complex ways. Progress appears to have been made in addressing age-related characteristics that put particular pressures on people in retirement, such as stabilizing or reducing the numbers in relative poverty. Similarly, measures designed to tackle age-based discrimination seem to be producing a cultural shift in the perceptions of older people. Those of us with interests in older people and work may not always appreciate these wider shifts in public attitudes.

We know that reducing avoidable adversity *and* increasing internal capacity strengthens coping during later life. This is why a primary prevention policy approach needs to increase education and access to learning opportunities; decision latitude over work; secure employment; safety within the home and within relationships; and good housing.

For older workers to remain in the workforce, new patterns of work and retirement are required (Reday-Mulvey 1999). A wide range of flexibility and options will probably result, including staggered, holiday blocks and part-time work. It will be interesting to observe which employers and in which sectors create these flexible patterns. Certainly, they have become apparent already in the retail sectors but not in all, and the retail sector itself is changing with online purchasing and large-scale outlets.

Conclusion

An ageing society and an ageing workforce test the capacity of employers and employees to work collaboratively for a number of reasons. The first is the complexity of older people's identities, wants and needs. The second is the heterogeneity of the workforce which, as Flynn and McNair describe in Chapter 3, contains people who are 'enthusiasts' about their work, those who find it 'stressful' in the context of other parts of their lives and those who are 'detached' or disillusioned by workplace attitudes to them. The third reason is the problematic and often unconscious meaning of older people as workers for younger colleagues and managers, in terms of the anxieties that this generates about ageing, capacity, disability and death. Finally, the multiple agencies involved in thinking about work in later life contribute to challenges for policy-makers and employers and workers in this area. In no other sector of work are responsibilities so diffuse and a European perspective permits UK thinkers to see that if issues are shared and values are held in common, then so too may be compromises and solutions.

References

Cuijpers, P., van Straten A. and Smit, F. (2006). *Improving Services and Support for Older People with Mental Health Problems*. London: Age Concern.

Meadows, P. and Volterra Consulting (2004) *The Economic Contribution of Older People*. London: Age Concern England.

Philipson, C. (2004) Work and retirement transitions: changing sociological and social policy contexts, *Social Policy and Society*, 3(2): 155–62.

Philipson, C., Scharf, T.I. and Smith, A.E. (2004) Poverty and social exclusion: growing older in deprived urban neighbourhoods, in *Growing Older: Quality of Life in Old Age*. (eds) A. Walker and C. Hagen Hennessy, Milton Keynes: Open University Press.

Reday-Mulvey, M. (1999) *Employment and Retirement: Gradual Retirement in Europe*. Geneva Papers September, Geneva: Geneval Association.

2 Working in later life: from yesterday's 'older worker' to tomorrow's 'key talent'

Sarah Harper[1]

Introduction

Until the past century, the term 'older worker' was synonymous not with the period prior to retirement but with ill health and low productivity, and it was this, far more than chronological age, which defined the term. Indeed, as late as the nineteenth century there are descriptions of men in their 40s defined as 'old workers' due to ill health and frailty working alongside energetic productive men in their late 60s or even 70s, to whom the term was not even applied. Male workers who made it into their 70s were often viewed as some of the most productive (Laslett 1995). In addition, and paradoxically, it is not the state of late-life work which defines retirement, but the growing emergence and redefinition of retirement which have over the past 50 years defined what it means to be an older worker. Thus, as the transition to retirement has moved chronologically earlier, so the age-based definition of 'older worker' has correspondingly shifted. The age of 45 or even 40, once considered the optimum time of a man's working life, has been seen over the past 20 years in many occupations in Europe as the commencement of falling productivity, decline and a period of late-life work prior to early retirement.

Such perceptions, however, appear set to change. Europe is now moving into a period of redefining late-life work as governments, employers and workers begin to come to terms with the implications of demographic ageing and the far-reaching implications these will have for institutions and individuals alike. There are now growing moves to recruit, retain and retrain that generation of men and women in their 50s and 60s who are increasingly being seen as essential to retaining Europe's economic competitiveness as the upcoming skills shortage washes across the region.

Defining and redefining the older worker

There is considerable historical evidence that work in some form continued throughout an individual's life until death (Thane 2000; McNicol 1998; Pelling and Smith 1991). For example, detailed analysis of old age and poverty in sixteenth-century Norwich (Pelling and Smith 1991) points out that less than two per cent were recorded as being unable to work. Older working men were recorded as undertaking a variety of labouring and non-labouring jobs – sweeping, pipe-filling, caretaking. Occupational segregation by gender appeared strict, and few men were noted as undertaking domestic tasks. While some older men were recorded as unemployed, it appeared unusual at this time for women to be labelled so. Indeed, women of child-bearing age were more likely to be unemployed than older women. This indicates that older women returned to the labour market once their child-rearing time had passed, rather than becoming minders and carers for grandchildren, or undertaking domestic work in the wider community – washing, cleaning, cooking – and caring for the sick both in homes and alms houses. Pelling and Smith (1991), for example, point out that women who were recorded as blind, lame and weak, still continued to knit, card and spin, noting the description of three widows, aged 74, 79 and 82 as being 'almost past work'. Similarly, older women were recruited by the authorities to teach children to knit, spin and weave (Willen 1988) and were specifically targeted to carry out certain occupations, such as keepers of the hospital. Pelling and Smith conclude that post-menopausal women were seen to have a positive value to society, which was lacked by men of a similar age. It is evident, however, that older men, in particular, shifted occupation as they aged (Thomas 1979), though they appeared to retain the occupational definition of their main life's work – carpenter, weaver, blacksmith, and so on.

A similar pattern of employment continued throughout the eighteenth and nineteenth centuries. Thane, writing about nineteenth-century England, describes how in urban areas:

> ... old factory hands [were] presented with a broom, shovel and wheelbarrow, old farm workers employed at stone-breaking and roadwork, old artisans in repair work, old miners working at odd jobs at the pithead, old dressmakers on rough sewing work, and old servants at daily work and charring ...
>
> (Thane 2000: 279)

Similarly, McNicol (1998) describes how the pattern of life for most people in rural communities was to go on working for as long as one was physically capable, moving to lighter or casual jobs, at progressively lower levels of pay until rendered completely unemployable by ill health, accident or disability.

During the twentieth century there was a slow withdrawal from employment at earlier and earlier ages, culminating in the emergence of mass retirement at a fixed age by the mid-1960s, and the growth of early retirement throughout the 1970s and 1980s. However, against this background, men in particular were also shifting into alternative occupations as in previous eras.

Consistent themes

The redefinition of older worker across the centuries has been overlain, however, by certain continuities, with older workers continually experiencing marginality, occupational cohort concentration, life course deskilling, perceived declining ability and late-life job transference. It is also clear that these continuities have been part of the experience of late-life work for skilled, professional and semi-skilled manual workers. However, though women's occupational evidence is not as prevalent as men's, it does seem that these continuities, while apparent in female working lives, have been stronger for men.

Marginality

Firstly, older workers have always been in a position of 'marginality'. During times of a tight labour market, older workers are more likely to be discharged in favour of younger workers. For example, during the interwar period unemployment was concentrated among older industrial workers (Thane 2000). Johnson (1994) argues that at this time both employers and trade unions conspired to preserve limited jobs for younger workers with family responsibilities. Indeed, there was an attempt early in the twentieth century to remove casual labourers (often older men) from the labour market in order to eliminate underemployment and low pay (Harris 1972). In addition, as Thane (2000) points out, older workers were concentrated in agriculture, with smaller groupings in sales work, clothing manufacture and labouring jobs; all occupations characterized by weak worker organizations, and thus vulnerable to employer-instigated redundancy. During times of labour deficit, older workers are targeted to undertake low-paid, casual and unregulated labour. This was clearly the case after the Second World War, for example, when older men and women were encouraged, alongside immigrants, to pick up a variety of unregulated, casual employment (Harper and Thane 1986, 1989). During times of wage increases, older workers are seen as expensive *vis-à-vis* their potential productivity and are either discharged or offered reduced hours. This has been represented in recent years by the debate concerning the marginal utility of older workers. As Casey et al. (1992) argues, with long-term contracts the wages of some older workers may simply exceed their marginal productivity, and it may be considered more cost effective for an organization to dismiss them, rather than extend equal opportunities to older workers.

Within the public sector the privatization of utilities and the introduction of compulsory competitive tendering have altered employment practices, in particular, threatening the opportunities for people aged over 50 (Burgess and Rees 1997). Similarly, within the private sector, the globalization of markets and the resultant increased competition have led to workforce reduction, which has particularly affected older workers. Leppel and Clain (1995) and Arrowsmith and McGoldrick (1997) highlight the selection of older workers for redundancy schemes, with the latter study revealing that older workers had been targeted for early retirement or redundancy packages in nearly 90 per cent of the organizations that were downsizing. A variety of other work has suggested that older workers are likely to be 'first out' in times of recession (Trinder 1989) and unlikely to be targeted for recruitment even in times of labour shortage (Thompson 1991; Lindley 1999). The exception to this is Sweden, with its tradition of 'last in first out', which has tended to penalize younger as opposed to older workers. Once unemployed, older workers are disproportionately less likely to find new work, so that older workers form a disproportionately higher proportion of unemployed workers in every EU country bar the Slovak Republic (Organization for Economic Cooperation and Development (OECD) 2006).

Occupational cohort concentration

Secondly, natural sectoral shifts in the economy mean that, unless there is a high level of inter-occupational mobility, workers find themselves employed in declining sectors as they approach later working life. At the turn of the century older workers in many European countries were concentrated in agriculture, this being the occupation which had been most readily available to them on entering the labour market in their youth. The subsequent contraction of agriculture from the late nineteenth century onwards accounted for most of the fall in economic activity rates of older men from the 1880s until the Great Depression of the 1920s (Johnson 1994). Thus, the decline in older male labour market participation in England, Wales, France and Germany, which occurred at the turn of the nineteenth/twentieth century, can almost all be accounted for through a general decline in agricultural employment, there being no significant corresponding increase in withdrawal of older men in industrial or service occupations (Thane 2000). Furthermore, employment rates of men in their 50s actually increased during 1891–1921 with the non-agricultural sectors providing alternative job opportunities for these men at this time (Thane 2000). Meanwhile, younger workers entered the new heavy industrial sector which had expanded throughout the nineteenth century, only to contract during the interwar years when these workers were themselves old.

There is a variety of contemporary evidence that older men, in particular, still tend to be employed in declining industries, underrepresented in new growth industries, and especially affected by reduced demand for unskilled workers (Jacobs et al. 1991; Trinder 1989; Gudgin and Schofield 1993). McKay and Middleton's (1998) secondary analysis of the United Kingdom (UK) Working Lives Survey 1994–5, for example, found concentrations of older men and women in manufacturing, suggesting that in terms of occupational profile by age, between three and four times as many men aged 65–69 were in unskilled occupations as those aged 45–49. Recent OECD figures (OECD 2001) demonstrate similar occupational concentrations by age, with the average age of male workers in engineering and manufacturing (a generally declining sector) now over 45, compared with the average age in the expanding information technology (IT) sector of under 35. This occupational differentiation by age is used by some in relation to the regional differentiation in decline in economic activity for older men. In the UK, for example, while nationally, between 1971 and 1991 male economic activity for those aged 50–69 fell by 19 per cent, this decline reached 23 per cent in northern England, but only by 16 per cent in the south east (Collis and Mallier 1996), in part reflecting different occupational opportunities in the two regions.

Life course deskilling

Thirdly, due to life-cycle effects, workers typically find themselves deskilled in late life. McNicol's (1998) comprehensive analysis of the history of British retirement between 1878 and 1948 reveals, for example, that from the 1880s onwards older workers were forced from the labour market due to technological intensification and an increasingly specialized segmented labour force. Technological developments in industry began to displace older workers who were judged unable to upgrade their skills or were surplus to requirements; older people were forced to retire because there were no jobs for them. Le Gros Clark (1968) makes a similar argument for the mid-twentieth century, when the increasing mechanization of many production processes was beginning to impact upon older workers. Older workers found the increase in pace required for some of these processes more difficult than younger workers. Thus, jobs requiring teams of workers operating at a pre-established rate had the highest retirement rate; conversely high-skilled occupations benefiting from experience had the lowest (Le Gros Clark 1968).

Such arguments pertain today, especially in IT sectors, exacerbated by the low level of training for those aged over 40 (Gibson 1993). However, while many argue that the requirement for new skills, particularly abilities in information and communication technologies, increasingly excludes older workers, especially men (Briscoe and Wilson 1991), others propose that technological innovation and flexible working patterns will increase opportunities for older workers (Lindley 1999; Casey et al. 1997), allowing them the possibilities of post-career employment (Arrowsmith and McGoldrick 1997). Harper (2000) has suggested that the inherent training component of new technological labour means that future cohorts of older workers will have experience of continual training and skills updating. For example, evidence from the USA suggests that workers in industries characterized by high rates of technological change will have later retirement ages as they tend to receive higher levels of on-the-job-training (Bartel and Sicherman 1993).

Perceived declining ability

There is a long-held view that older workers are unproductive. As Harper (2006) points out, there has been a variety of historical evidence along these lines from the early twentieth century to the present, and stereotypical attitudes towards older workers appear to have shown little improvement since research carried out in the 1950s by, for example, Kirchner and Dunnette (1954), Le Gros Clark (1959) and Belbin (1958). Yet, 50 years ago, there was ample evidence that older workers were seen as a valued component of the workforce, to which they made an active and valuable contribution (Harper and Thane 1986, 1989). While there were changes in capacity with age, these could be overcome through retraining and adaptation of the work environment (Welford 1958; Meier and Kerry 1976; Fleischer and Kaplan 1980). Furthermore, an age-integrated workforce was perceived to be a versatile workforce (Belbin 1958; Le Gros Clark 1959).

Slow work speed, low adaptability, particularly to new technologies, low trainability, low skills uptake and being too cautious, are stereotypes which appear to arise consistently in surveys (Casey et al. 1992; Taylor and Walker 1994; Crimmins and Hayward 1997). Forte and Hansvick's (1999) Survey of Chamber of Commerce Members Pacific North West, for example, found that while older workers were rated more highly in terms of academic skills, ability to get along with co-workers, willingness to take directions, work ethic, productivity and supervisory skills, younger workers were rated more highly in terms of computer skills, stamina and energy, flexibility, and ability to learn quickly, characteristics which Arrowsmith and McGoldrick (1996) describe for the UK in terms of qualitative and quantitative characteristics. Older workers retained the former, high quality of service, pride in job, cheerfulness, reliability, while younger workers exhibited so-called quantitative characteristics – fast pace of work, trainability and adept at handling new technology.

Yet, there is little practical evidence to support the views that people aged over 50 are consistently less able to perform modern economic activity than those younger (Lindley 1999), while Warr (1994) points out that generally variations within age groups far exceed those across age groups. Indeed, a recent OECD (2006) report shows that worker productivity does not decline with age as diminishing abilities are compensated for by acquired skills and experience.

Late-life job transference

As we saw earlier, there has historically been a move in later working life, particularly for men, from a full-time, typically lifelong, occupation to more casual, intermittent and typically less skilled work, at the end of male working lives. This continued to be documented throughout the twentieth century as an alternative to the state of full-time retirement, or while men were waiting to reach pensionable age. During the labour shortages of the 1960s, the transference of older workers into 'alternative' occupations was seen as preferable to redesigning their current occupations or working environments. There is considerable British evidence, for example, that job transfers were common for men over 55, with one-fifth transferring in their 60s (Harper and Thane 1986, 1989). Such jobs were not only those that were less physically demanding, but also ones in which speed and dexterity were not required.

In addition, we may already be seeing a more composite transition from full-time economic activity to full-time retirement. This may include periods of unemployment, employment and 'retirement', and the growing use of second career or 'bridge jobs'. Early retirement may be for some a transition from the first to a second career (Labour Force Survey and ONS Retirement Survey in Disney et al. 1997) indicating that these workers have an increased tendency to be in self-employment. These sets of data may reflect the increased levels of opportunities for self-employment due to the accumulation of social and economic capital at these ages. There is also evidence that this group is moving at great rates into small businesses, which may increasingly form the transitional bridging jobs between work and retirement. Evidence from a recent global survey of 40–80-year-olds suggests that workers across the world would like more flexible working in their later lives, including career changes in their 50s and more part-time work (Leeson and Harper 2006).

From yesterday's 'older worker' to tomorrow's 'key talent'

The last decade has seen a growing government awareness of the importance of retaining Europe's older workers. With a current employment rate of only 41 per cent for those aged 55–64 (33 per cent for women) (Eurostat 2007), an emerging European skills shortage and a looming pension burden, encouraging older workers to stay active with the labour market is a key EU aim. The concept of 'flexicurity' has become the new EU policy objective: developing and sustaining flexible contracts, active labour market policies, lifelong learning and modern social security systems. This is seen as a response to the need to improve the adaptability of workers and firms to rapidly changing labour markets and job segmentation. Evidence continually shows that the long-term trend of increasing institutional support for age-structured employment careers has halted. Younger people are less likely to spend their careers in jobs that provide greater rewards and security for longer tenure with a firm. Older workers will hold the expectation of far more variable patterns of career endings, plus the possibility that more non-career jobs will be available. This has in part been encouraged by changes towards the service sector. Here employers are more likely to have contingent and part-time employment arrangements. Similarly, within-firm changes are occurring. In order to cope with increasing competition and technological change, some employers are keeping a smaller proportion of employees in career employment, and more in contingent employment, which allows greater adaptability.

Furthermore, the attitudes and experiences of older people today are not necessarily those of the future. Younger cohorts, currently in early and midlife, will have very different education, labour market and health experiences. They are already growing accustomed to a less rigid labour market (Gallie 1998), with greater access to part-time and flexible working patterns, and the need for continual skills updating and retraining. These individuals may have different aspirations in later life, and the financial incentives and disincentives for economic employment will undoubtedly have changed. Alongside this is growing evidence from the United States of America (USA) (Manton 2000) that these cohorts will be healthier, and that this cohort effect is likely to continue into old age. The economic and social attitudes towards late-life employment and retirement are thus likely to be different, possibly very different, for these younger cohorts who are approaching late-life work and retirement decisions over the next three decades.

One can argue that just as we saw a cyclical labour market trend which mirrored the demographic patterns in the last quarter of the twentieth century, a similar cyclical trend is emerging today. The emphasis on retaining older workers at times of youth labour shortages was replaced by a negative view of older people as a younger labour force emerged, so the predicted downfall in younger people entering the labour market over the next 20 years will in itself lead to the retention of older workers and a more integrated workforce. However, as we have seen in this chapter and others in this book, there are now considerable complexities in the system and attitudes are firmly entrenched in some sectors, both in relation to the characteristics of older workers and in the attractions of early retirement. It may need effective intervention by governments to counterbalance these. The policies against age discrimination may be only part of the required strategy to integrate older people back into the workforce. Rather, governments may need to introduce more targeted schemes, such as the Scandinavian early retirement and transitional retirement schemes. These were introduced in the four Nordic countries in the late 1980s and early 1990s as a means of enabling older workers to withdraw from full-time employment. Now they are being considered as a means not to remove older workers but to retain them through allowing a flexible withdrawal from full-time employment. Denmark, for example, has recently reformed its scheme which allows transitional early retirement through raising the number of hours allowed to be worked and the lifetime insurance contributions required to be paid in order to qualify for the scheme in an attempt to encourage more participation in the labour market (Jensen 1999). The Finnish gradual retirement scheme was introduced in 1987 for public and 1989 for private workers partially to increase flexibility on retirement.

Another policy option is to encourage employers to hire and retain older workers through the use of subsidies. Here the argument is that the only way to break down ageist stereotypes and to create conducive working environments and business structures for an integrated workforce is for employers to see that such workforces provide good business practice. There already exist several such subsidy schemes in Europe. French companies hiring unemployed people aged 50 or above can take advantage of the *Contrat Initiative Emploi* (contract to promote employment), a subsidy which reduces the employers' social security contributions. It is paid indefinitely if the person is disabled or has been unemployed for more than one year. Germany has an integration subsidy, the *Eingliederungszuschusse*, that corresponds to 50 per cent of wages for those hiring long-term unemployed people aged over 55. Sweden's Special Employment Subsidies programme encourages employers to recruit persons aged above 57 who have been unemployed for at least two years. However, as is clear, all these are targeted at long-term unemployed older people, rather than at older workers in general. Furthermore, of course, there is the possibility that such age-targeted programmes would be challenged under full age discrimination legislation.

The Norwegian model is an example of a more holistic approach. In 2001 the government and social partners (employers and trade unions) in Norway signed a tripartite agreement on a more inclusive workplace. The employer must set up systems to systematically address the problem of ill health and declining functions, and when an employee is unable to continue their job due to sickness or ill health, the employer is obliged, in collaboration with the authorities, to supply training so the person can be qualified for another job in the company, clearly an easier task within large companies. In return, the employee must inform the employer about changing functional capacity, agree to a dialogue with the employer about necessary changes in work tasks, participate in whatever training is considered necessary, and cooperate with the employer on adapting the workplace as necessary.

This is important because it lays out the key elements of a long-term strategy for encouraging and facilitating an integrated workforce: adapt the financial incentive and benefit system to encourage the retention of the older workforce; and adapt the work environment to create a more flexible inclusive workplace. This will undoubtedly bring benefits to all workers across the life course; training and education for all including continual skills upgrading; increase dialogue between employers and employees so that all workers are seen as individuals, and not numbers defined by their age, enabling all workers to plan and adapt for all life course transitions.

Flexible inclusive workplace

The past 20 years have seen increasing recognition within OECD countries of the need to improve both physical and psycho-social work environments. The OECD report provides a template for developing inclusive age-integrated working environments based on flexibility and individualization (OECD 2003a). The working environment should be adapted through work rotation, reorganization of work tasks and ergonomic improvements, and employees should feel they have control over their own work situation wherever possible. In particular, all workers should have flexibility in their working-time arrangements, including the possibility of part-time work at times of life course need.

Training and education

Furthermore, as has already been discussed, the inherent training component of new technological labour means that future cohorts of older workers will have experiences of continual training and skills updating. Supplemented by vocational and lifelong learning, adult education and training, this will significantly enhance the employability of older people (OECD 2001) and address national skills shortages, particularly in the health and social care sectors (see Chapters 6 and 11). Some European countries already operate study leave schemes allowing employees to return to full- or part-time education or training (OECD 2003b). It is important that such education and training are targeted, built on previous experiences and skills, and are properly evaluated. Far more research and evaluation of the effectiveness of different types of lifelong learning and training are required from a business stance. However, the general impact of education at all ages on health and well-being should not be underestimated.

Dialogue: planning for late-life work

This element may well in the long term prove to be the most crucial. One of the key areas of concern expressed by European employers in relation to age discrimination is managing the departure of older workers. Whether this is a convenient front behind which to hide, is a real business issue, or is symptomatic of the tremendous change in attitudes towards late-life work and older people which have occurred over the past 25 years, is unclear. The key here is dialogue between employer and employee. One of the drivers discussed earlier for the introduction of mass retirement at a fixed age was the increasing bureaucraticization and administration of the workplace. Faced with these complex procedures, employers found the ability to remove set known numbers of workers each year and thus replace and train new workers as a convenient administrative tool. This was before the development of highly sophisticated and competent human resource tools, teams and departments. Indeed, the professional body of this group is committed to the removal of age discrimination in employment because it is seen to be wasteful of talent and harmful to both individuals and organizations (Chartered Institute of Personnel and Development (CIPD) 2004). Given the tremendous success highlighted earlier of early and pre-retirement training courses in persuading an entire cohort that retirement was a positive step, similar planning for late-life work courses and training programmes aimed at highlighting the benefits, necessity and potential for the individual of late-life work will also play a key role here, and should form a crucial component of government strategies. Furthermore, the concern that employees whose performance declines towards the end of their careers will be subjected to the indignity of performance/capability procedures will disappear when such performance/capability procedures are routine for all employees across the life course.

Conclusion

As a recent Manpower Report concluded: 'The first priority of today's employers should be forecasting and workforce planning for the future, when much of today's key talent will retire and there will be few available candidates to replace them' (Manpower 2007: 24).

Both recent employers' surveys by Manpower (Manpower 2007) and the HSBC Future of Retirement Survey (Leeson and Harper 2006) found a slow but growing awareness of the need to retain 'a company's DNA' (Leeson and Harper 2006), though interestingly this was generally highest in the fast-growing Asian economies than in Europe (Manpower 2007) despite the high numbers of young people in Asian countries. Indeed, it is clear that the majority of European Human Resource professionals have yet to engage with the reality of future skills shortages (Manpower 2007). Of highest importance, however, is the ability of employers and national governments to understand the work-life balance of older workers. This will require the introduction of a high level of flexible working patterns into today's labour markets, to allow for the conflicting family-work demands of these generations, and to respond to the increasing psycho-social recognition by individuals of the importance of and desire to control their later life work years. Highly skilled older European workers will increasingly be able to choose their own mix of flexible/part-time work supported by relatively high-level pension benefits. Employers need to put in place strategies to recruit, retrain and retain these individuals. Lower-skilled older workers will either be unable to retire due to low-pension benefits, or will desire to remain within the labour market for social and psychological reasons (Leeson and Harper 2006). Here national government policies have to be implemented to ensure that these individuals can also be active and contributory for as long as they are able. Many European national-funded pension schemes will be unable to fulfil their obligations given the predicted large numbers of older individuals who will be drawing down pension provisions in a system with too few economically active contributors to support them. Given that a percentage of older men and women will simply be unable to work in later life due to ill health and frailty, governments should ensure that all older people that can make an active contribution to the economy and society are fully enabled to participate.

Note

1 I would like to acknowledge the assistance of Sue Marcus in the research for and planning of this chapter.

References

Arrowsmith, J. and McGoldrick, A.E. (1996) HRM service practices: flexibility, quality and employee strategy, *International Journal of Service Industry Management*, 7: 46–62.

Arrowsmith, J. and McGoldrick, A.E. (1997) A flexible future for older workers. *Personnel Review*, 26: 258–73.

Barham, C. (2002) Patterns of economic activity among older men, *Labour Market Trends*, 110: 301–10.

Bartel, A.P. and Sicherman, N. (1993) Technological change and retirement decisions of older workers. *Journal of Labor Economics*, 11: 162–83.

Bassanini, A. and Scarpetta, S. (2001) Does human capital matter for growth in OECD countries? *Economics Letters*, 74: 399–402.

Belbin, E. (1958) Methods of training older workers. *Ergonomics*, 1: 207–11.

Burgess, S. and Rees, H. (1997) Transient jobs and lifetime jobs: dualism in the British Labour. *Oxford Bulletin of Economics and Statistics*, 59: 309–28.

Casey, B., Lakey, J. and White, M. (1992) *Payment Systems: A Look at Current Practice*. Sheffield: England Employment Department.

Casey, B., Metcalf, A. and Millward, N. (1997) *Employers Use of Flexible Labour*. London: Policy Studies Institute.

Chartered Institute of Personnel and Development (CIPD) (2004) *Age and Employment*. London: CIPD.

Collis, C. and Mallier, T. (1996) Third age male activity rates in Britain and its regions, *Regional Studies*, 30(8): 803–9.

Crimmins, E.M. and Hayward, M.D. (1997) What can we learn about competence at the older ages from active life expectancy?, in W. Schaie, S. Willis and M.D. Hayward, (eds) *Social Structural Mechanisms for Maintaining Competence in Old Age*, pp. 1–22. New York: Springer.

Disney, R., Grundy, E. and Johnson, P. (1997) *The Dynamics of Retirement: Analysis of the ONS Retirement Survey*. Washington, DC: Department of Social Security.

Eurostat (2007) *EU Labour Force Survey Annual Results 2006*. Brussels: Eurostat.

Fleischer, D. and Kaplan, B.H. (1980) *Work and Retirement: Policy Issues*. Los Angeles, CA: University of Southern California Press.

Forte, C.S. and Hansvick, C.L. (1999) Applicant age as a subjective employability factor: a study of workers over and under age fifty. *Journal of Employment Counseling*, 36: 24–34.

Gallie, D. (1998) *Equal Opportunities for Women and Men in Europe? Eurobarometer 44.3 – Results of an Opinion Survey*. Luxembourg: Office for Official Publications of the European Communities.

Gibson, C. (1993) The four baby booms, *American Demographics*, 15: 36–40.

Gould, R. and Solem, P.E. (2000) Change from early exit to late exit: a Finland/Norway comparison. Paper presented at the *COSTA Meeting, Ageing and Work*, Rome, 13–14 April.

Gudgin, G. and Schofield, A. (1993) The emergence of the north–south divide and its projected future, in R. Harrison and M. Hart (eds) *Spatial Policy in a Divided Nation*. London: Jessica Kingsley/Regional Studies Association.

Harper, S. (2000) Ageing 2000 – questions for the 21st century, *Ageing & Society*, 20: 111–22.

Harper, S. (2006) *Ageing Societies: Myths, Challenges and Opportunities*. London: Hodder Arnold.

Harper, S. and Thane, P. (1986) The social construction of old age in post-war Britain – 1945–1965. Working paper, Social History Series. Goldsmiths College, University of London, London.

Harper, S. and Thane, P. (1989) The consolidation of 'old age' as a phase of life, 1945–65, in M. Jefferys (ed.) *Growing Old in the Twentieth Century*, pp. 43–61. London: Routledge.

Harris, J. (1972) *Unemployment and Politics: A Study in English Social Policy, 1886–1914*. Oxford: Clarendon Press.

Hellerstein, J.K., Neumark, D. and Troske, K.R. (1999) Wages, productivity and worker characteristics: evidence from plant level production functions and wage equations. *Journal of Labor Economics*, 17: 409–46.

Henretta, J.C. (1994) Recent trends in retirement. *Reviews in Clinical Gerontology*, 4: 71–81.

Jacobs, K., Kohli, M. and Rein, M. (1991) Testing the industry-mix hypothesis of early exit, in M. Kohli (ed.) *Time for Retirement: Comparative Studies of Early Exit from the Labor Force*, pp. 67–96. Cambridge: Cambridge University Press.

Jensen, P.H. (1999) *Activation of the unemployed in Denmark since the early 1990s*. Welfare of Workfare? Report for the Centre for Comparable Welfare Studies. Aalborg: Aalborg University.

Johnson, P. (1994) The employment and retirement of older men in England and Wales, 1881–1981, *Economic History Review*, 47: 106–28.

Kirchner, W.K. and Dunnette, M.D. (1954) Attitudes toward older workers. *Psychology*, 7: 257–65.

Laslett, P. (1995) Necessary knowledge: age and ageing in the societies of the past, in D.I. Kertzer and P. Laslett (eds) *Aging in the Past: Demography, Society, and Old Age*. Berkeley: University of California Press.

Le Gros Clark, F. (1959) *Age and the Working Lives of Men*. London: Nuffield Foundation.

Le Gros Clark, F. (1968) *Pensioners in Search of a Job*. London: Nuffield Foundation.

Leeson, G. and Harper, S. (2006) *The Future of Retirement Report: What Businesses Want*. London: HSBC.

Leppel, K. and Clain, S. (1995) The effect of increases in the level of unemployment on older workers. *Applied Economics*, 27: 901–6.

Lindley, R.M. (1999) Population ageing and the labour market in Europe. *Rivista Italiana di Economia, Demografia e Statistica*, LIII: 167–92.

Loscocco, K. (2000) Age integration as a solution to work-family conflict. *Gerontologist*, 40: 292–300.

Manpower (2007) *The New Agenda for and Older Workforce: Retain/Retire*. Milwaukee, USA: Manpower Inc.

Manton, K. (2000) Gender differences in the cross-sectional and cohort age dependence of cause-specific mortality: the United States, 1962 to 1995, *Journal of Gender-Specific Medicine*, 3: 47–54.

McKay, S. and Middleton, S. (1998) *Characteristics of Older Workers: Secondary Analysis of the Family and Working Lives Survey*. London Department for Education and Skills (www.dfee.gov.uk/research/report45.html).

McNicol, J. (1998) *The Politics of Retirement in Britain, 1878–1948*. Cambridge: Cambridge University Press.

Meier, E.L. and Kerr, E. (1976) Capabilities of middle-aged and older workers: a survey of the literature, *Industrial Gerontology*, 3(3): 147–55.

Ministry of Labour (1945–55) Unpublished memos, UK Ministry of Labour, London.

Organization for Economic Cooperation and Development (OECD) (2001) *Ageing and Income: Financial Resources and Retirement in 9 OECD Countries*. Paris: OECD.

Organization for Economic Cooperation and Development (OECD) (2003a) *Ageing and Employment Policies – Sweden*. Paris: OECD.

Organization for Economic Cooperation and Development (OECD) (2003b) *Employment Outlook*. Paris: OECD.

Organization for Economic Cooperation and Development (OECD) (2006) *Ageing and Employment Policies – 'Live Longer, Work Longer'* (www.oecd.org/dataoecd/32/50/36218997.pdf, Paris).

Pelling, M. and Smith, R.M. (1991) *Life, Death and the Elderly: Historical Perspectives*. London: Routledge.

Quinn, J.F. and Kozy, M. (1996) The role of bridge jobs in the retirement transition: gender, race and ethnicity, *Gerontologist*, 36: 363–72.

Takala, M. (1999) The part-time pension programme in Finland Paper presented at the *Active Strategies for an Ageing Workforce Conference*, Turku, Finland, 11–13 August.

Taylor, P. and Walker, A. (1994) The ageing workforce: employers' attitudes towards older workers, *Work, Employment and Society*, 8: 569–91.

Thane, P. (2000) *Old Age in English History: Past Experiences, Present Issues*. Oxford: Oxford University Press.

Thomas, K. (1979) Age and authority in early modern England. *Proceedings of the British Academy*, 42: 206–48.

Thompson, M. (1991) *Last in the queue? Corporate employment policies and the older worker*, report No. 204. Brighton: Institute of Manpower Studies.

Trinder, C. (1989) *Employment After 55*. London: National Institute for Economic and Social Research.

Warr, T. (1994) Age and employment, in H.C. Triandis, M.D. Dunnette and L.M. Hough (eds) *Handbook of Industrial and Organizational Ppsychology*, 2nd edn, pp. 485–550. Palo Alto, CA: Consulting Psychologists Press.

Welford, T.A. (1958) *Ageing and Human Skill*. Oxford: Oxford University Press.

Willen, D. (1988) Women in the public sphere in early modern England: the case of the urban working poor. *Sixteenth Century Journal*, 19: 559–75.

3 What would persuade older people to stay longer in work?

Matt Flynn and Stephen McNair

In the United Kingdom (UK), as in most developed countries, there is a growing interest in older workers' willingness to remain economically active longer. Real retirement ages declined over the last quarter of the twentieth century; but the trend now appears to have reversed, and in 2006 reached 64.2 years for men and 61.8 for women (the highest since records began in 1984). The UK is ahead of its European neighbours in keeping older people economically active (High Level Group chaired by Wim Kok 2004), the government still has the ambition to increase the number of older workers (over 50) by one million (Department for Work and Pensions (DWP) 2005). Although most of the emphasis has been on keeping people economically active until they reach retirement age (e.g. meeting the Lisbon targets, UK pension rules to disallow retirement before 55), there is a growing interest in work after retirement age.

Much of the debate over work in later life has centred on the sustainability of both the State and private pension systems. Because over a third of firms have closed or are planning to close their defined benefit pension schemes to new entrants, and the State Pension continues to fall behind average earnings, if left unchecked, retirement will be unaffordable to the current working-age population. However, the current cohort of workers who are leaving the labour market are still part of the 'golden age' of retirement, and it will be some years until the 'pension time bomb' fully hits. The more immediate drivers are labour shortages and skills demands. As unemployment falls, employers are increasingly looking for ways to encourage their older workers to stay in work longer in order to fill skills gaps and maintain workforce levels. Employers in regions such as London and the south east, and sectors such as retail have been particularly eager to delay retirement for their older workers. Government has also recognized that continued economic growth depends on an increase in older people's economic activity, and a modest growth in labour participation could remedy both the short-term skills shortage and longer-term pension crisis (Meadows 2004).

Under the European Union (EU) Employment Equality Directive of 2000 all EU countries are establishing age discrimination legislation, and in the UK this took effect in October 2006. A key element of the British Regulations is the outlawing of compulsory retirement ages before the new national Default Retirement Age of 65 (a majority of employees still have retirement ages in their contracts of employment, although a majority of firms – mainly smaller ones – do not). However, the Regulations also introduce a statutory 'right to request' to stay longer than the employer proposes, and the employer is obliged to consider such requests, though he or she can ultimately insist.

The Regulations have been heavily criticized for giving the final say about whether a worker can delay retirement to the employer. The government is, however, hoping that introducing the right will increase the number of requests, and that, when approached by older workers, employers will see the merit of agreeing. This 'light touch' (Department of Trade and Industry (DTI) 2005, para 6.3.3) approach is meant to facilitate dialogue between older workers and their employers not only about whether working life should be extended, but also more importantly, the kind of work which would be carried out and the plan for eventual retirement. The 'right to request' extended work was modelled on existing law giving the right to request flexible working to parents of young children, and the government pointed to that law's success in generating a change in workplace culture.[1] Data from the annual work-life balance survey indicates that over three-quarters of requests for flexible work were granted (Hooker et al. 2006).

Without overlooking the considerable leverage that employers have in deciding how and when older workers retire, it is worth considering whether workers who are close to retirement would be amenable to extending work. Although the onus is on employers to inform employees who are due to retire that they can ask to stay longer, workers who want to delay retirement are expected to initiate discussion about how work will be designed once they pass normal retirement age. Who will want to remain in paid work? What kind of work could be requested?

These questions have been considered from a number of different angles, but one of the key issues is how older workers view work in general and their current jobs, and what influence this has on their inclination to work beyond retirement age. This was one of the issues which the Centre for Research on the Older Worker (CROW) sought to investigate in a postal survey of older workers in 2004, and which forms the subject of this chapter.

Attitudes towards work and retirement – the literature

In recent years, research interest in older workers' attitudes towards work and retirement has grown, with two major programmes, the Economic and Social Research Council's (ESRC) 'Growing Older' programme (Walker 2004) and the Joseph Rowntree Foundation's 'Transitions after 50' (Hirsch 2003) programme making major contributions. The ESRC's New Dynamics of Ageing programme was also expected to contribute to this area, although it did not fund any projects on the older workforce in its first (2005) round.

Much of the focus has been on the transition from work to retirement, and the push and pull factors which encourage workers to retire early from work (Humphrey et al. 2003). Push factors which have been identified include health problems (accompanied by poor management); caring responsibilities; career plateaus; age discrimination; and employers' use of early retirement to manage restructuring and downsizing. Pull factors include financial security; expectations of older workers; and the view of retirement as an earned reward.

Commentators have often suggested that it would be desirable to replace the traditional 'cliff edge' retirement (from full-time work to full-time retirement at one point in time) with a more gradual approach. 'Bridging jobs' (usually with less responsibility or fewer hours which individuals take on to smooth the transition from full-time work to retirement) (Lissenburgh and Smeaton 2003) are popular with older workers, even when accompanied by extended working life. However, opportunities for gradual retirement are rare and workers who seek them face institutional barriers. (Loretto et al. 2005). Bridging jobs, such as portfolio jobs, can be less secure, particularly if the worker is employed on an *ad hoc* basis (Platman 2003). As with opportunities for early retirement, the choices people make reflect their gender, job class, education and attitudes.

It is self-evident (though often ignored in policy discussions) that older workers are not a uniform group, and if government and employers want to encourage workers to stay in work longer, they need to understand how different groups of older people view work and retirement. The simplest and oldest of these attempts is Titmuss's 'two nations' of privileged workers with much choice over retirement and the subjugated who have retirement thrust upon them. However, Titmuss's model was designed for a very different labour market, and he never specifically considered the issue of work in later life (in his day work to state pension age (SPA) was normal and retirement brief). Since then attempts have been made to produce a more refined model (AARP 2002; Barnes et al. 2004; Employers Forum on Age 2005; McNair et al. 2004). Clustering can be based around attitudes towards and motivation to work qualifications, occupation and sector, gender and social class. The

CROW surveys have sought to clarify these issues and explore the possibility of a more relevant model which would be of greater use to policy-makers and researchers.

The CROW survey

In 2003, CROW conducted a survey of people aged 20–69 years looking at experience with job transitions (McNair et al. 2004). The survey was carried out by adding five questions to three rounds of the Office of National Statistics' monthly Omnibus Survey. The survey generated responses from 5,402 people (1,136 of them aged over 50) giving information about the frequency, causes and outcomes of job change. One of the five questions asked respondents whether they would consider working after retirement, and 77 per cent of those in work (including 79 per cent of those over 50) said that they were willing to do so. This finding was striking and controversial, although it has since been confirmed by studies by the Employers Forum on Age (Employers Forum on Age 2005) and Age Concern/Heyday (Age Concern 2006), while HSBC found a similar pattern of attitudes in a study of retirement in 14 countries (HSBC 2005). It is also notable that interests in working longer increased with age, with those over 50 years of age much more likely to consider this than those in their 20s and 30s.

In order to enrich the findings of the Omnibus Survey, a much more detailed questionnaire was distributed to respondents aged over 50 who agreed to be followed up. This questionnaire asked 44 questions (38 of them to those in work). A total of 401 people responded, of whom 195 were economically active while 32 of these considered themselves 'retired but still in paid work'.

Attitudes to work

The survey asked 17 questions, in each offering five levels of response, from 'strongly agree' to 'strongly disagree'. The questions are shown in Table 3.1.

Overall, this represents a remarkably positive set of attitudes to work among older people, and should offer some encouragement to government. Almost seven in ten workers who are in work now would miss it if they were to retire. Most find their work satisfactory; their colleagues enjoyable to work with; and feel that their employers respect their experience and work. Those who define themselves as 'retired but still in paid work' are even more positive about their work. However, there remains a significant minority of older workers who are dissatisfied with their work. For any given factor,

Table 3.1 Attitudes to work

	Strongly agree	Agree
Work content		
My job is enjoyable	16	61
My job makes good use of my skills and abilities	27	49
My job is mundane	2	16
I do not feel my work makes a contribution to society	3	13
Work colleagues		
I enjoy working with my colleagues	21	58
My friendships with people at work are important to me	26	54
I spend a lot of time helping younger colleagues	6	38
Employer		
My experience is valued by my employer	17	47
My employer is encouraging me to stay in work as long as I can	7	33
My employer does not value the work I do	2	9
Work-life balance		
My job is well suited to my personal circumstances	18	60
I find it hard to balance home and work commitments	3	25
Finance		
I need to work to increase my pension	17	42
I need to work in order to keep employment benefits	4	23
I need to work to support others	14	23
I could afford to retire now	3	18
Views on work		
I would miss working if I retired today	24	45

between a fifth and a third of workers express dissatisfaction. Strongest dissatisfaction is reflected in workers' attitudes towards their employers. Around a third of workers do not feel that their experience is valued by their employers, and only a minority think that their employers are encouraging them to stay in work.

It has been suggested that finance may not be a critical factor in decisions on the timing of retirement, partly because retirement finance is such a complex issue that many people cannot calculate the likely impact, and choose to take early retirement offers which seem superficially attractive (Hirsch 2003). However, the CROW survey suggests that finance plays a more important part in older workers' decisions to stay in work than previous research suggests (perhaps because of changes to pension schemes during the intervening period). A large majority of respondents said that they could not afford to retire now, although this is not surprising, given that the sample ranged in age from 51–70, and a significant proportion were still in their early to mid-50s. However, this was also true for people in their mid- to late 60s as well as the 60 per cent of those who consider themselves retired from their main jobs, but are still in work, which suggests that finance is a major motivation for continuing after 'normal retirement age' for some. Finance does, however, seem to play a more important role in decisions on whether to continue in work, and many who work past retirement age do so in order to maintain their accustomed lifestyles.

One might assume that the generally positive views show that those who like work stay longer, while those who are dissatisfied with their jobs leave. This is not the case. The 194 respondents who were already retired were asked to rate their *last* jobs with the same criteria. Retired people were as positive in responding to the questions on job content, their former colleagues, their former employers and work-life balance. They were, however, more likely to say that retirement is now affordable; and less likely to miss work.

Attitudes to retirement

Just over half of those surveyed said that they have no plans to retire. As they approach SPA, workers are more likely to set a planned retirement date, but three-quarters of those over SPA (60 for women, 65 for men) have no plans to retire. Table 3.2 shows the reasons older workers gave for the dates they have chosen to retire.

Of those who have set a retirement date, most feel that they have exercised some choice over when. A third say that they will retire at the age they want to, while over a quarter say that they will work until they feel they can afford to retire. Although only 30 per cent of respondents say explicitly that they plan to retire 'when they reach SPA', two-thirds of men who name a date say that they expect to retire at 65 and two-thirds of women expect to retire at 60.

Surprisingly few workers – fewer than one in ten – say that they expect to retire when they reach their employers' retirement age (multiple choices were allowed). Given the controversy over the government's decision to set a default retirement age and the Confederation of British Industry's intensive lobbying for employers' continued right to set a mandatory retirement age, few workers see it as a significant factor when deciding when to retire. If government does decide to abolish mandatory retirement in 2011 (when it has promised to review the default retirement age) or if the European Court of Justice compels it to do so earlier, it does not appear that it will have a strong impact over workers' attitudes (which is not to say that abolition will not affect how employers manage retirement).

Table 3.2 Reasons for choosing a retirement date (%)

This is the age I want to retire	34
This is the state pension age	30
To enjoy retirement as soon as I can afford to	28
I need to work longer to top up my pension	14
This is the age my financial commitments reduce	14
This is my company's specified retirement age	9
This is the age my partner plans to retire	6
I have the option of retiring early and want to take it	4
I have other commitments	4
I want to do voluntary work	3
I have no plans to retire at present	52

Multiple responses were allowed

In the Omnibus survey, respondents were asked whether they would consider working after retirement age, and the responses were surprisingly positive, with 80 per cent agreeing. To clarify the evidence the question was slightly rephrased in the postal survey by asking older workers if they *would like* to be in paid work after retiring from their main jobs. As earlier, there was strong interest from those in employment in continuing in work after normal retirement age.[2] A quarter said that they would definitely want to continue in work; another quarter said they would probably like to do so; and a further 20 per cent said that they might 'if the right job came along'.

Most of those who would like to, or would even consider paid work after retirement only want to do so on a flexible or part-time basis. Fifty-six per cent would like to work part time, and 34 per cent would work occasionally; but only 8 per cent would consider continuing work full time. It is clear that what is sought is a gradual transition into retirement (at whatever age) rather than a deferring of 'cliff edge' retirement.

Attitudes to government policy

Older workers broadly support government's aim to extend working life, although they distrust its motives. Remarkably, a significant minority (29 per cent) felt that because people are living longer, it is reasonable to raise the minimum retirement age. There was near unanimous agreement that people should be able to continue in work 'so long as they are fit and capable' (94 per cent) and most older workers felt that their collective skills are not being put to best use (90 per cent). A majority (57 per cent) considered that the economy needs older workers to be encouraged to work longer in order to remain productive.

However, when asked about what drives government policy, three-quarters felt that it is motivated by a desire to reduce the tax and pension burdens on younger people and that public policy is a threat to the right to retire.

Most older workers who were surveyed believe that more flexible ways of working (87 per cent) and opportunities to work closer to home (57 per cent) are needed to persuade people to defer retirement. However, two-thirds also see the need for more training and information about job opportunities; and 38 per cent said that career and life planning would help.

How attitudes to work affect retirement plans

One of the biggest unexplored questions is how older workers' views on their jobs impact on their expectations for work after retirement. Given that the survey found both generally positive attitudes towards work and a general willingness to consider work after retirement, some relationship between the two might be expected. But which aspects of work have the biggest impact? What positive experiences would persuade people to work longer?

To get some insight into this question, a regression analysis was conducted using the 17 questions on work as independent variables; and responses to the question 'Would you like to be in paid work after you retire from your main job' were used for the dependent variable. As Table 3.3 shows, five factors appeared to be significant. Job content, work-life balance, financial considerations such as pensions and benefits, and an expectation that work would be missed in retirement each incline workers to want to stay in paid work longer.

Table 3.3 Factors inclining a desire to stay in paid work after retirement from main job

	Standardized coefficients		F	Sig.
	Beta	Std. error		
My job is enjoyable	0.41	0.14	9.08	0.00
I find it hard to balance home and work commitments	–0.38	0.13	8.97	0.00
I need to work to increase my pension	0.29	0.13	5.22	0.00
I would miss working if I retired today	0.30	0.12	6.28	0.00
I need to work in order to keep employment benefits	0.35	0.13	7.89	0.01

If we take work enjoyment, work-life balance, pensions and missing work (pensions and benefits intercorrelate) along with willingness to work after retirement from main job, a two-step clustering can be carried out to identify three groups. Each has a different set of characteristics in terms of experience in work and attitudes towards work and retirement. They are described here as the 'enthusiasts', 'detachers' and 'over-stressed'. The age profile of the three groups is similar (see Table 3.4 which shows the three groups characteristics).

Table 3.4 Group attitudes to work

	Enthusiasts	**Detachers**	**Stressed**
Work content			
My job is enjoyable	100	60	78
My job makes good use of my skills and abilities	94	72	90
My job is mundane	0	44	23
I do not feel my work makes a contribution to society	3	28	25
Work colleagues			
I enjoy working with my colleagues	100	78	97
My friendships with people at work are important to me	100	84	90
Employer			
My experience is valued by my employer	91	40	100

	Enthusiasts	Detachers	Stressed
My employer is encouraging me to stay in work as long as I can	53	36	62
My employer does not value the work I do	9	30	3
Work-life balance			
My job is well suited to my personal circumstances	97	86	69
I find it hard to balance home and work commitments	12	38	52
Finance			
I need to work to increase my pension	59	54	91
I need to work in order to keep employment benefits	44	32	20
I could afford to retire now	12	14	24
Views on work			
I would miss working if I retired today	82	66	58
Wanting to work after retirement			
Yes	58	30	52
Maybe	18	41	0
No	24	27	48

Enthusiasts, as the name implies, are the most contented with work and are most likely to want to continue in work longer. A significant proportion (58 per cent) of this group would like to carry on in full-time work. They are the most keen to see mandatory retirement age abolished. They are also the most keen to change jobs or seek a promotion within their firm. They are also the least likely to have set a retirement date as yet. This group thinks that training and career advice could most encourage older workers to extend working life.

Two-thirds of the *detachers* are women. Although the majority are still motivated by the same factors as the enthusiasts, all of them are weaker. They are less likely to find their work challenging, and more likely to feel undervalued by their employers (although it is unclear which problem causes which). This group is most likely to have caring responsibilities; and the most likely to have had their last job transition imposed upon them (e.g. redundancy). They are most likely to have suffered discrimination in the workplace (33 per cent against 18 per cent across all groups). This group is more likely to see flexible and home-working options as effective in motivating older workers to stay longer and social motivation seems to be weaker (perhaps because their social relationships are based in the home or community rather than the workplace). Only 30 per cent would like to work after retirement, but a further 41 per cent could be persuaded to, perhaps reflecting never having been asked.

The *stressed* have enjoyable jobs and are respected by their colleagues, but they have difficulty balancing home and work commitments. A third would like to work shorter hours, and a quarter spend a lot of their working days travelling. This group is predominantly men and more likely than the other two to be in managerial and professional jobs. A fifth has caring responsibilities, who, unlike the detatchers, have not downshifted in order to balance home work responsibilities. The *stresseds'* last job change resulted in more responsibility, a need for more skills and longer hours. The most interesting aspect of this group is that it is evenly divided between those who would clearly want, and definitely do not want, to work after retirement. Given previous evidence that high-job status workers have the greatest flexibility in later life transitions, the overstressed probably are exercising the most choice out of the three groups, but half of them are, to use Vickerstaff's phrase, choosing to jump off the cliff (Vickerstaff 2006).

Discussion

The CROW survey shows that older workers, in general, find work fulfilling, enjoy working with their colleagues, feel valued and would miss work if they stopped today. Most say that they want to continue in work after what they expect to be their retirement date. These statements are true for a majority in all three groups identified above. Although most older workers say that they want to stay in work longer, we know that few actually do. The survey gave some clues about why the gap between aspiration and experience exists.

First, although part-time and flexible work is, conceptually, an attractive alternative to retirement, many older workers do not see it as a feasible option for them. This is particularly the case for people identified here as the stressed. Arguably, this group has the greatest autonomy in work, but many find downshifting or reducing hours either unattractive or unfeasible. One of the biggest barriers may be job design, with members of this group in jobs which have traditionally been exclusively full time. Managerial jobs have been particularly difficult for reduced hours, even for the large retailers who have run high-profile campaigns to recruit older workers (see McNair and Flynn 2005, case study 3 'Supermarket', p. 102).

Employers who want to encourage older workers to consider flexible working as an alternative to retirement will need to be more proactive than the new law prescribes in designing reduced hours jobs which are attractive to older workers. If older workers (and as importantly their line managers) are unable to see how they can continue work with reduced hours, it is difficult to see many making requests.

In contrast, those who have made adjustments to work in order to accommodate family responsibilities (identified here as the detached) – often earlier in their careers when raising children – leave work before they want to because they are in jobs which are not fulfilling and their potential contribution is unrecognized by their employers. This might be an obvious commentary on the gender gap in work and effect which child-rearing has on career patterns. However, it does also point to the risks which employers can take in ignoring skills needs and career expectations of older workers and allowing them to coast in work leading up to retirement. People who feel undervalued by their employers, and do not sense that they are making a contribution in the workplace may drift into retirement without considering possibilities for working longer. This group may need a greater and earlier intervention than the right to request envisions. Clearly, the opportunity to work longer would need to be made in unison with chances to develop and participate in work that is challenging and fulfilling.

The third group – the enthusiasts – seems to have found the right balance between flexibility and job fulfilment, and this group seems the most likely to request to stay in work longer. However, they feel that career advice, job opportunities and training are as, if not more, important incentives for staying in work longer as opportunities to reduce working hours. Bridging the transition from work to retirement may therefore not be the objective for many who ask to stay in work longer, and extended working life may be seen as a new stage in their careers. This presents a challenge to employers who may have a more limited view on work after retirement. The new law gives employers scope to fix periods for post-retirement work (but employees still have the right to request to stay on when such periods lapse), and some older workers may feel dissatisfied with the chance to wind down in their jobs within fixed contract periods.

The new regulations may have a catalytic effect on how employers and employees consider work and retirement. The dramatic increase in the real retirement age (after decades of decline followed by stabilization) probably reflects changes at the lower end of the spectrum (e.g. employers closing early retirement options in light of changes to pension rules). However, the prospect of a new right to request extended work has likely encouraged some workers to think about delaying retirement. As more older workers ask to stay in work longer, employers could find it easier to accommodate requests. Nevertheless, older workers will need active support from their employers to consider extended work options. Employers will need to demonstrate how work can be flexible, valuable and rewarding to encourage requests from older workers to be generated.

Notes

1 Although research suggests that the success of the right to request flexible working conceals workers' reluctance to ask for alternative work arrangements when they expect to be denied. (Fagan et al. 2006)

2 'Retirement age' was not defined in the questionnaire, and it is clear that different people have different notions of what 'retirement' means.

References

AARP (American Association for Retired People) (2002) *Staying Ahead of the Curve*. Washington, DC: AARP.

Age Concern (2006) *Age Concern Launches 'Heyday' to Meet the Needs of the Modern Retiree*. Age Concern: London.

Barnes, H., Parry, J. and Taylor, R. (2004) *Working After State Pension Age: Qualitative Research*, Research Report No. 208. London: Department for Work and Pensions.

Department of Trade and Industry (DTI) (2005) *Equality and Diversity, Coming of Age: Consultation on the Employment Equality Regulations 2006*. London: DTI.

Department for Work and Pensions (DWP) (2005) *Opportunity Age*. London: The Stationery Office.

Employers Forum on Age (EFA) (2005) *Attitude not Age: A Wake Up Call About the UK's workforce*. London: EFA.

Fagan, C., Hegewisch, A. and Pillinger, J. (2006) *Out of Time: Why Britain Needs a New Approach to Working-time Flexibility*. London: Trades Union Congress.

Hirsch, D. (2003) *Crossroads After 50: Improving Choices in Work and Retirement*. York: Joseph Rowntree Foundation.

Hooker, H., Neathey, F., Casebourne, J. and Munro, M. (2006) *The Third Work-life Balance Employees' Survey*. London: Department of Trade and Industry.

HSBC (2005) *The Future of Retirement in a World of Rising Life Expectancies*. London: HSBC.

Humphrey, A., Costigan, P., Pickering, K., Stratford, N. and Barnes, M. (2003) *Factors Affecting the Labour Market Participation of Older Workers*, Research Report No. 200. London: Department for Work and Pensions.

Kok, W. (chair) (2004) *Facing the Challenge: The Lisbon Strategy for Growth and Employment*. Luxembourg: Office for Official Publications of the European Communities.

Lissenburgh, S. and Smeaton, D. (2003) *Employment Transitions of Older Workers: The Role of Flexible Employment in Maintaining Labour Market Participation and Promoting Job Quality*. Bristol: The Policy Press.

Loretto, W., Vickerstaff, S. and White, P. (2005) *Older Workers and Options for Flexible Work*. Manchester: Equal Opportunities Commission.

McNair, S. and Flynn, M. (2005) *The Age Dimension of Employment Practice: Employer Case Studies*. London: Department of Trade and Industry.

McNair, S., Flynn, M., Owen, L., Humphreys, C. and Woodfield, S. (2004) *Changing Work in Later Life: A Study of Job Transitions*. Guildford, University of Surrey: Centre for Research into the Older Workforce (CROW).

Meadows, P. (2004) *The Economic Contribution of Older People*. London: Age Concern.

Platman, K. (2003) The self-designed career in later life: a study of older portfolio workers in the United Kingdom, *Ageing and Society*, 23: 281–302.

Vickerstaff, S. (2006) 'I'd rather keep running to the end and then jump off the cliff', Retirement, Retirement Decisions: who decides? *Journal of Social Policy*, 35(3): 455–72. Available online (www.journals.cambridge.org/action/displayAbstract;jsessionid=056FD06A644AE4EF13593CF8CAE10685.tomcat1?fromPage=online&aid=449177#>).

Walker, A. (2004) The ESRC *Growing Older* research programme, 1999–2004, *Ageing and Society*, 24(5): 657–74.

4 Are European older workers on the verge of a 'golden age' of employment opportunities?

Philip Taylor

Introduction

This chapter considers the changing status of older workers in the European labour market, examining the rolling back of passive public policy responses in the form of early exit pathways in favour of a new emphasis on activation. It considers the strength of a recent reversal in employment rates and asks whether older workers can look forward to employment choice and job security or whether they are being used as a reserve army of labour, to be deployed on certain fronts while continuing to be excluded or withdrawn from others.

A changing employment landscape

Until recently, early retirement dominated the employment landscape for older workers in Europe. As the 1980s got under way, a pre-existing trend towards early retirement gathered pace as recessions and restructuring of industry occurred in western Europe. In many countries governments implemented early retirement pathways; in some disability benefit systems were (mis)used and firms sometimes utilized occupational pension schemes to pay out older workers. Youth unemployment was the major public policy concern and attempts at job creation via the removal of those aged over 50 a key response. The opening up of the markets of the central and eastern European economies subsequently led to pressures on older workers here too. The meaning of this 'early retirement' for older workers has long been a subject of debate, but is seems clear that there were marked variations in the extent to which there was an element of 'voluntarism' among those exiting. It is the case that for many 'early retirement' could be more accurately described as a kind of unemployment. Moreover, where older workers had previously experienced at least a modicum of certainty about their date of retirement, that had now gone. The result has been the breakdown of the three-phase model of the life course: education, work and rest. 'Socially assigned' economic inactivity has made the last stage of life 'unforeseeable and uncertain' (Guillemard and Argoud 2004: 168). Guillemard argues that the passage from work to retirement has undergone a profound shift, with 'an increasing number of in-between, usually unstable, statuses between work and retirement' (1997: 451). Even those from the higher management strata have not been immune, although they remain generally better off than the rest. On top of this was a social consensus about the value of early retirement to individuals, organizations and economies. It needs to be stressed that, with few exceptions, the direction of pressure on older workers was almost entirely in the direction of a truncation of working lives. The strength of this consensus almost exactly mirrors that of today, but, of course, in reverse.

On the back of concerns about future labour supply and about the future sustainability of pensions systems bought about by population ageing and decline in fertility rates, since the beginning of this decade European and national policy-makers have striven to bring early retirement to a halt and to put in place measures that will push out the boundaries of when work finally ceases. The debate has shifted from one of protecting the young to 'active ageing'. In a short period of time a remarkable body of literature has emerged which seeks to undermine the case for early retirement and to position older workers as the solution to employers' labour supply needs.

On the face of it, European governments and business have much to be concerned about. As can be seen in Table 4.1, among men aged 50–64, employment rates quickly fell in the last two decades of the twentieth century, the result of industry restructuring and as many governments in western Europe implemented programmes of early retirement with the support of both business and trade unions which sought to exchange older workers for young labour market entrants. Europe compares poorly with Japan and the United States of America (USA), although it is notable that there is considerable variability in the European scene, with Sweden, for instance, having an employment rate that exceeds the USA and compares favourably with Japan. Elsewhere, however, the situation is much less favourable.

Table 4.1 Employment/population ratios for men, 55–64 age group over time (%)

Country	2005	2004	2003	2002	2001	1995	1990	1983
Austria	41.3	38.9	40.2	39.5	37.9	40.8	–	–
Belgium	41.3	39.3	38.7	35.1	35.1	34.5	34.3	47.7
Czech Republic	59.4	57.2	57.5	57.3	52.6	50.6	–	–
Denmark	66.8	69.3	68.0	64.2	63.0	63.4	65.6	63.1
Finland	52.5	51.5	51.4	48.3	46.7	34.9	46.3	51.4
France	43.8	44.5	44.9	44.2	34.9	38.4	37.0	50.4
Germany	53.6	50.7	47.1	47.2	46.4	48.8	52.0	57.4
Greece	58.8	56.4	58.3	55.3	54.6	58.9	58.4	68.8
Hungary	40.6	38.4	37.9	35.4	34.1	27.1	33.3	–
Ireland	65.7	64.7	64.8	65.1	64.6	59.1	59.5	69.2
Italy	42.7	42.2	42.8	41.2	40.4	42.3	51.9	55.3
Japan	78.9	78.1	77.4	76.8	77.5	80.8	80.4	95.2
Luxembourg	38.3	38.0	39.1	37.6	35.3	35.1	42.9	37.8
Netherlands	–	56.3	56.1	56.0	50.5	31.5	44.5	50.5
Poland	37.9	36.0	36.8	35.8	37.1	42.5	44.3	–
Portugal	58.1	59.1	61.6	61.2	61.3	58.9	65.0	69.1
Slovak Republic	47.9	43.8	41.0	39.1	37.6	–	–	–
Spain	59.7	58.9	59.3	58.6	57.9	48.0	57.3	65.2
Sweden	–	71.6	71.1	70.8	69.6	64.4	74.5	73.9
UK	65.7	65.4	64.9	62.0	61 6	56.1	62.4	62.6
USA	67.0	66.0	65.6	66.3	66.0	63.6	65.2	65.2
EU-15	53.1	52.1	51.8	50.7	48.6	–	52.3	–
EU-19	51.8	50.7	50.6	49.4	47.5	–	51.1	–
EU						47.2		58.5

Notes:

UK 1983 refers to 1984

Hungary and Poland 1990 refers to 1992

For 1990 and 1983 there is no data for EU-15 or EU-19, refer to EU

Data for years 2005–2002 come from 2006 OECD

Data for years 2001–1990 come from 2005 OECD

Data for the year 1995 come from 1999 OECD

Data for the year 1983 come from 1997 OECD

(–) appears where there is no information for that country for that year

Also apparent in Table 4.1 is a general shift in favour of older male workers in recent years. The improvement is fragmented. Some countries have seen little or no improvement, while elsewhere a clear upward movement is noticeable. It is also clear that while some nations' employment rates among older workers are drawing level with or exceeding those for previous decades, others are falling far short. It would also not be appropriate to describe this upward trend as dramatic, at least in recent years.

Table 4.2 Employment/population ratios for women, 55–64 age group over time (%)

Country	2005	2004	2003	2002	2001	1995	1990	1983
Austria	22.9	19.3	20.7	19.2	17.4	18.3	–	–
Belgium	23.0	21.2	17.7	16.7	15.6	12.7	9.4	11.8
Czech Republic	31.0	29.4	28.4	26.0	23.2	20.5	–	–
Denmark	52.9	54.2	53.1	49.9	49.8	36.1	42.4	39.1
Finland	52.7	50.4	48.5	47.3	45.1	34.0	39.7	44.1
France	37.6	36.8	35.9	34.6	26.7	28.9	25.0	30.4
Germany	37.6	33.0	30.9	30.1	29.4	27.0	22.4	24.0
Greece	25.8	24.0	25.3	24.2	22.7	23.8	24.0	25.2
Hungary	26.8	25.0	21.8	17.6	14.9	9.2	14.3	–
Ireland	37.4	34.0	33.5	30.7	28.4	19.4	18.2	18.9
Italy	20.8	19.6	18.5	17.3	16.2	13.1	15.2	14.6
Japan	49.4	48.6	47.5	47.1	47.3	47.5	46.5	45.1
Luxembourg	24.8	22.0	20.9	18.1	14.4	13.2	13.7	14.1
Netherlands	–	33.2	30.8	29.7	28.0	14.0	15.8	12.5
Poland	21.4	21.0	21.5	21.1	22.0	26.3	27.8	–
Portugal	43.7	42.5	41.8	41.9	40.2	33.6	31.7	31.8
Slovak Republic	15.7	12.6	11.2	9.6	9.8	–	–	–
Spain	27.4	24.6	23.4	22.0	21.8	17.6	18.0	19.7
Sweden	–	67.4	66.8	65.9	64.3	59.5	64.7	57.4
UK	48.2	47.3	46.3	44.5	43.2	39.3	36.7	33.4
USA	55.1	54.3	54.5	53.2	51.7	47.5	44.0	39.4
EU-15	35.0	32.9	32.4	31.0	29.0	–	24.3	–

Country	2005	2004	2003	2002	2001	1995	1990	1983
EU-19	33.4	31.5	31.0	29.6	27.8	–.	24.3	–
EU						25.6		25.0

Notes:

UK 1983 refers to 1984

Hungary and Poland 1990 refers to 1992

For 1990 and 1983 there is no data for EU-15 or EU-19, refer to EU

Data for years 2005–2002 come from 2006 OECD

Data for years 2001–1990 come from 2005 OECD

Data for the year 1995 come from 1999 OECD

Data for the year 1983 come from 1997 OECD

(–) appears where there is no information for that country for that year

The situation for women is equally diverse (see Table 4.2). There is a general upward trend, substantial in some countries, rather more modest in others. Again, there are marked differences between nations. Rates among some northern European nations clearly exceed those for Japan and are roughly comparable with those for the USA.

It should be noted that taking such a broad age sweep as this disguises marked differences by age in employment rates in many European countries. France is an example of a pronounced fall after the age of 60. Even so, if different age groups are considered, as in Table 4.3, then it is notable that while employment rates drop off after age 60, among the 60–64 age group too, rates in most European countries demonstrate an upward trend. Interestingly, among the over-65s, a rather more mixed picture emerges.

Table 4.3 Employment/population ratios men and women between 2000 and 2006

			Year						
			2000	2001	2002	2003	2004	2005	2006
Country	Sex	Age group							
Austria	Men	55 to 59	60.0	61.0	63.4	65.8	62.5	62.4	66.0
		60 to 64	16.4	17.2	17.0	16.4	16.6	19.6	21.1
		65+	4.3	4.9	3.8	3.7	3.7	4.9	5.5
	Women	55 to 59	24.4	26.8	31.8	35.3	32.8	38.0	40.9
		60 to 64	7.7	8.6	7.8	7.4	7.0	8.1	9.9

			Year						
			2000	2001	2002	2003	2004	2005	2006
		65+	1.6	2.2	1.7	1.7	1.2	1.7	2.2
Belgium	Men	55 to 59	52.0	50.4	50.9	52.3	54.4	54.2	51.8
		60 to 64	18.1	19.2	16.5	21.2	19.1	23.8	20.7
		65+	2.2	2.3	2.0	2.4	2.4	2.2	2.8
	Women	55 to 59	24.1	25.9	26.0	26.7	31.6	32.5	32.4
		60 to 64	7.0	5.4	6.4	6.8	7.8	10.5	10.6
		65+	1.1	0.7	0.6	1.0	0.5	0.8	1.0
Czech Republic	Men	55 to 59	71.8	73.4	76.6	76.6	76.9	78.5	78.4
		60 to 64	23.5	23.2	29.3	30.2	30.1	33.8	34.9
		65+	6.7	6.6	6.4	6.3	5.9	6.1	6.5
	Women	55 to 59	30.9	31.6	36.2	39.6	42.4	45.8	47.9
		60 to 64	11.2	12.1	12.1	13.4	12.5	12.2	12.7
		65+	2.3	2.1	2.2	2.2	2.2	2.2	2.4
Denmark	Men	55 to 59	79.7	77.3	80.9	80.7	83.7	82.7	84.8
		60 to 64	37.8	43.3	43.3	49.9	51.0	47.3	51.7
		65+	3.7	6.4	8.2	7.0	7.9	9.4	8.4
	Women	55 to 59	64.3	69.5	69.8	70.8	72.5	74.8	74.8
		60 to 64	23.4	24.2	24.1	27.5	29.7	26.3	29.3
		65+	1.6	3.2	2.5	3.2	1.9	2.3	2.8
Finland	Men	55 to 59	58.9	62.3	64.5	65.2	64.7	63.3	65.9
		60 to 64	26.8	28.2	28.7	31.5	31.3	35.6	39.2
		65+	6.3	6.2	6.2	7.6	7.4	7.3	7.7
	Women	55 to 59	59.9	63.8	65.5	66.7	67.0	67.3	68.9
		60 to 64	20.1	22.4	23.5	23.7	27.0	31.0	35.0
		65+	1.6	1.6	2.5	2.0	2.4	3.2	4.4
France	Men	55 to 59	60.5	62.8	64.8	64.1	62.6	61.1	60.5
		60 to 64	14.7	15.0	16.7	17.8	17.9	17.5	18.3
		65+	1.9	1.7	1.8	1.9	1.8	1.7	1.6
	Women	55 to 59	47.2	48.3	50.2	51.2	51.8	52.4	52.7
		60 to 64	12.8	12.5	14.5	14.9	15.2	15.7	16.7
		65+	0.9	0.9	0.9	0.8	0.9	0.9	0.8
Germany	Men	55 to 59	66.3	67.6	68.8	68.3	70.0	71.6	72.4
		60 to 64	27.7	29.0	30.3	30.4	34.2	35.9	38.2
		65+	4.4	4.4	4.3	4.4	4.4	5.0	5.0
	Women	55 to 59	47.1	48.7	50.6	51.8	53.5	55.3	56.9
		60 to 64	12.5	13.8	14.7	15.1	16.5	20.7	22.2
		65+	1.5	1.8	1.8	1.8	1.6	2.2	2.3
Greece	Men	55 to 59	69.2	69.7	68.4	71.7	69.1	70.8	71.4
		60 to 64	43.9	41.7	42.1	43.3	41.6	43.7	44.1

			Year						
			2000	2001	2002	2003	2004	2005	2006
		65+	8.3	7.6	7.8	8.0	6.8	6.9	7.3
	Women	55 to 59	29.7	27.4	28.6	30.4	28.3	31.2	31.6
		60 to 64	19.9	18.8	19.7	19.8	19.0	20.0	21.3
		65+	2.7	2.7	2.3	2.4	2.0	1.9	2.0
Hungary	Men	55 to 59	49.6	51.4	52.8	55.2	54.0	56.6	58.6
		60 to 64	11.6	13.1	14.4	16.8	20.1	20.9	19.2
		65+	3.8	3.1	3.4	3.8	4.3	4.2	4.2
	Women	55 to 59	20.0	23.2	28.3	35.1	39.8	41.8	42.6
		60 to 64	5.0	5.5	6.0	7.3	9.0	9.6	8.9
		65+	1.8	1.3	1.5	2.0	1.9	1.4	1.6
Ireland	Men	55 to 59	71.8	73.5	73.4	72.7	73.2	71.6	74.0
		60 to 64	52.6	53.6	54.2	54.5	53.5	58.2	57.5
		65+	14.7	14.2	14.8	14.0	13.6	14.6	14.4
	Women	55 to 59	34.0	34.9	37.0	40.8	41.5	45.1	47.4
		60 to 64	19.2	20.5	22.8	24.1	24.4	27.5	30.9
		65+	2.9	2.9	3.0	3.3	3.0	3.2	4.2
Italy	Men	55 to 59	51.5	51.6	53.1	55.3	54.0	55.5	56.4
		60 to 64	30.0	29.5	29.6	30.6	29.1	27.6	28.0
		65+	5.8	6.0	6.0	5.8	5.9	5.9	6.1
	Women	55 to 59	23.0	24.5	26.3	27.5	29.5	31.2	32.0
		60 to 64	7.8	8.5	8.9	9.9	9.1	9.1	9.8
		65+	1.5	1.5	1.5	1.5	1.2	1.1	1.2
Japan	Men	55 to 59	90.0	89.5	88.8	88.8	89.4	89.6	89.6
		60 to 64	65.1	64.6	64.0	64.7	65.4	65.9	67.1
		65+	33.0	31.7	30.3	29.0	28.4	28.7	28.4
	Women	55 to 59	57.0	56.5	56.2	56.7	58.0	58.4	58.6
		60 to 64	37.8	37.7	37.5	37.5	38.4	39.0	39.0
		65+	14.2	13.7	13.2	12.9	12.8	12.6	12.8
Luxembourg	Men	55 to 59	56.5	55.3	53.3	57.9	56.9	56.7	..
		60 to 64	16.5	12.3	18.7	17.5	14.9	14.4	..
		65+	2.3	1.1	2.4	2.1	1.1	1.0	..
	Women	55 to 59	20.9	22.7	27.3	30.2	34.2	36.3	..
		60 to 64	12.5	5.6	8.1	10.0	8.3	11.0	..
		65+	1.2	0.5	0.5	0.9	0.4	0.4	..
Netherlands	Men	55 to 59	68.6	72.2	74.4	73.4	73.6	74.3	75.4
		60 to 64	26.7	25.5	30.7	30.1	30.8	29.0	32.3
		65+	5.5	5.3	6.1	6.2	6.4	7.2	7.8
	Women	55 to 59	37.9	38.6	42.4	42.2	45.2	47.3	50.7
		60 to 64	11.2	12.6	13.2	14.6	16.2	17.3	19.7

			Year						
			2000	2001	2002	2003	2004	2005	2006
		65+	1.5	1.4	1.9	2.1	1.8	2.0	2.0
Poland	Men	55 to 59	46.6	47.8	44.3	45.6	43.7	44.9	46.0
		60 to 64	27.1	25.7	25.5	24.6	24.1	25.6	25.3
		65+	11.8	11.5	9.9	8.9	9.0	9.0	8.0
	Women	55 to 59	28.5	29.5	28.3	27.5	26.4	26.6	23.6
		60 to 64	14.9	14.5	12.9	13.6	13.3	13.1	11.8
		65+	5.0	4.7	4.5	4.4	4.2	3.9	3.3
Portugal	Men	55 to 59	70.6	69.4	71.3	70.5	67.3	66.9	65.9
		60 to 64	53.3	52.7	50.5	52.3	49.3	47.4	48.9
		65+	25.0	25.6	25.7	26.0	25.5	24.6	24.6
	Women	55 to 59	46.2	44.6	48.6	49.6	49.3	49.9	48.2
		60 to 64	35.3	35.7	35.1	33.9	34.6	36.4	36.7
		65+	13.2	13.8	14.1	13.7	12.4	13.2	13.2
Slovak Republic	Men	55 to 59	56.2	61.6	62.2	65.5	65.9	68.7	68.7
		55 to 64	35.4	37.6	39.1	41.0	43.8	47.9	49.9
		60 to 64	9.8	8.3	11.0	11.3	15.4	20.2	22.7
		65+	1.7	1.8	1.8	2.0	2.0	2.1	1.9
	Women	55 to 59	15.7	15.0	15.2	18.1	19.6	23.6	28.8
		60 to 64	3.1	3.8	3.3	3.4	4.4	6.1	6.4
		65+	0.4	0.4	0.3	0.7	0.7	0.8	0.7
Spain	Men	55 to 59	68.8	69.8	70.5	70.7	70.6	71.3	72.5
		60 to 64	40.0	43.8	44.0	45.5	44.8	46.2	46.6
		65+	2.5	2.6	2.4	2.3	2.3	3.1	3.3
	Women	55 to 59	24.7	26.8	27.5	28.7	30.6	34.7	36.3
		60 to 64	15.1	16.0	15.7	17.1	17.7	19.1	20.1
		65+	0.9	0.9	0.9	0.9	1.0	1.1	1.1
Sweden	Men	55 to 59	79.7	80.3	81.1	79.4	79.9	82.0	81.6
		60 to 64	51.6	54.9	56.7	60.1	61.5	61.0	62.9
		65+	14.7	13.5	14.3	14.5	12.5	14.5	13.8
	Women	55 to 59	76.0	77.2	77.1	76.9	77.1	77.3	77.5
		60 to 64	45.0	47.1	50.9	53.7	55.4	55.0	56.2
		65+	6.3	5.8	5.6	6.1	6.2	5.7	6.6
UK	Men	55 to 59	70.8	72.6	72.9	73.8	74.6	75.1	75.5
		60 to 64	47.3	48.4	48.4	53.2	53.4	53.7	54.5
		65+	7.7	7.0	7.6	8.7	8.6	8.9	9.7
	Women	55 to 59	55.9	57.0	58.1	61.3	61.0	62.3	62.7
		60 to 64	25.3	27.1	27.8	27.2	29.7	30.3	32.3
		65+	3.4	3.0	3.6	3.6	3.9	4.4	4.5
USA	Men	55 to 59	75.3	74.8	74.7	74.2	74.5	75.0	75.2

		Year						
		2000	2001	2002	2003	2004	2005	2006
	60 to 64	53.5	54.6	55.1	54.5	54.8	56.2	57.0
	65+	17.1	17.2	17.2	17.8	18.3	19.1	19.8
Women	55 to 59	59.9	60.0	61.6	63.0	62.6	63.4	64.8
	60 to 64	39.2	41.4	42.5	43.7	43.7	44.3	45.6
	65+	9.1	9.3	9.5	10.2	10.7	11.1	11.4

Source: OECD Stats.

While early retirement took hold, population ageing coupled with low fertility began to radically alter the composition of the European population. The populations of the developed economies are the oldest in the world. Europe will be most affected by population ageing, with the proportion of people aged 60 or over increasing from 20 per cent to 35 per cent by 2050. Southern Europe is the world's region with the oldest population – 22 per cent in 1998 – and is predicted to increase to 39 per cent by 2050. In 1998, Italy had the world's oldest population, followed by Greece, Japan, Spain and Germany. By 2050 Spain will have the world's oldest population, followed by Italy. After Europe and Japan, the other areas particularly affected by ageing are, in decreasing order, North America, Oceania, Asia and Latin America and the Caribbean (Auer and Fortuny 2000). The paradox between retiring earlier and living longer is clear and has alarmed European policy-makers who wish that Europe could be as competitive as the USA and Japan, and it is to the rapid turnaround in the ways older workers are viewed that this chapter now turns.

Policy reform

The closure of early retirement pathways and the imperative of extending working lives have been a preoccupation of European and national policy-makers over the last decade. European targets agreed at the Barcelona and Stockholm European Councils concerning employment rates for older workers and increasing the average age of retirement, the Equal Treatment Directive, a vast range of official reports and numerous research studies funded by the European Commission and other European bodies have sought to establish the conditions for European member states to put in place their own measures. These have been forthcoming, although progress has been fitful, and there has been considerable resistance at times from trade unions wishing to retain members' rights to retire early and employers wanting to retain the right to choose when and how to dismiss older workers. While it is clear that public policy-makers have, on the whole, accepted the need for reforms aimed at prolonging working lives, this also has its limits. Strong efforts to encourage and support all older workers to work later and to protect them if they do, have not so far been implemented. Policy-makers, partly due to fierce opposition from employers, have baulked at the notion of 'age free' employment, as it is sometimes known.

Can public policy support older workers to compete in modern economies or are they to be left largely at the mercy of market forces? The position of the EU and its members is predicated on the notion that governments can turn the early retirement tide. Unfortunately, there is much uncertainty regarding the effectiveness of public policies targeting older workers. It is known, for instance, that those transitioning from employment programmes are prone to occupational downshifting and struggle then to move to higher level positions (Taylor 2006). It is also the case that they continue to be underrepresented in programmes offering learning and training opportunities. Added to this, although flexible working is widely canvassed as giving older workers the opportunity to make a gradual transition to retirement, such measures as have been implemented might be viewed as *de facto* early retirement schemes (Frerichs and Taylor 2005), or at least those working longer being offset by those retiring earlier as a result of their availability. In one recent Finnish case, take-up appeared to have depended on the government lowering the age of entry (Taylor 2002). It is not easy to see how these could be viewed as successful examples of flexible retirement, yet this is frequently put forward as a credible option for allowing people to work later and in easing the transition to retirement. In fact, contrary to what is commonly argued by a number of commentators, far from winding down to retirement, many older workers would like to work more hours. The latest European Working Conditions Survey asks those working part time whether they would like to work more hours. An analysis carried out for this chapter demonstrates that, taking all respondents aged over 50 together (Tables 4.4 and 4.5), approximately a fifth classified as such would have liked to increase their working hours. If a finer age categorization is used, then between the ages of 50 and 59, it can be seen that a sizeable minority were dissatisfied with their working hours; approximately one-quarter wanting them to increase. Even among the 60–64 age group, while satisfaction with working hours was high overall, approximately one-tenth (13 per cent) wanted them to increase.

Table 4.4 Would you like to work ... ?

	Frequency	Per cent
Full time	193	12.3
More hours but not full time	124	7.9
The same number of hours	968	61.5
Less hours	157	10.0
DK/no opinion	86	5.5
Refusal	46	2.9
Total	1574	100.0

Source: European Working Conditions Survey 2005, author's analysis.

Table 4.5 Would you like to work ... ?

			Age group				Total
			50–59	55–59	60–64	65+	
Full time		Count %	88	74	24	7	193
			16.9	15.8	7.9	2.5	12.3
	More hours but not full time	Count %	58	41	18	7	124
			11.1	8.8	5.9	2.5	7.9
	The same number of hours	Count %	288	284	200	196	968
			55.2	60.8	65.6	70.0	61.5
	Less hours	Count %	49	38	36	34	157
			9.4	8.1	11.8	12.1	10.0
	DK/no opinion	Count %	22	18	22	24	86
			4.2	3.9	7.2	8.6	5.5
	Refusal	Count %	17	12	5	12	46
			3.3	2.6	1.6	4.3	2.9
Total		Count %	522	467	305	280	1574
			100	100	100	100	100

Source: European Working Conditions Survey 2005, author's analysis.

Thus, flexibility should not be viewed, as it so often is, as a one-way street towards retirement. An appropriate policy response would consider how to provide older workers with a degree of choice about their labour market participation. Altogether, while early exit was a hugely successful invention, it has proved, perhaps unsurprisingly, harder to reinvent retirement. Coming up with an appropriate policy mix that promotes working later is proving elusive.

Challenges ahead

As previously mentioned, employment rates for older workers are increasing in much of Europe. Does this mean that their prospects are getting brighter? Compared with past times this does indeed appear to be the case. Previously, older workers have fared poorly, even during periods of economic growth. Perhaps the difference now is that, whereas previously industry could turn to reservoirs of young people as markets recovered, this may no longer be the case. But considerable caution is required here. There is evidence that current economic growth explains much of the improvement in older workers' fortunes but cohort effects seem to explain much of the rest (Hotopp 2005), and if older workers are working later as it seems, this seems to be going against the wishes of European employers who still do not seem to be too interested in them. Although commentators and public policy-makers envisage a scene of labour-starved industry welcoming older workers to fill the gap left by absent young labour market entrants, other scenes may be played out. Certainly, despite the apparently obvious logic of ageing populations meaning ageing workforces, at least in the minds of many observers, employers continue to see things differently, with older workers not featuring strongly in plans for tackling issues of labour supply (Henkens et al. 2006).

There are also examples from a recent study completed by this chapter's author, which looked at practices in over 100 European organizations of employers seemingly unconcerned by the implications of low fertility and population ageing, deliberately removing older workers from jobs, using familiar methods, in response to increasing global competition. For instance, in 1999, Belgian company *Barco* participated in a regional project called 'Life Time Employability'. The organization considered it important to foster 'replenishment' periods of training during the careers of their employees. The company's workforce is ageing and some older workers find it hard to keep up, despite intense training programmes, and the company has promoted employee cases known as 'beacons' as examples for other workers (e.g. flexible working hours arrangements, part-time work, downshifting and outplacement). However, in 2004, the company restructured some of its divisions. Blue-collar workers aged 50 and over were offered a 'Canada Dry-arrangement', which consists of unemployment benefits and a lump sum paid by the employer. Most took advantage of the offer. Another company example is Swedish company *Rapid's* initiative to recruit older workers in the 1990s. Since then it has reduced the size of its workforce.

Dismissal regulations protect older employees, meaning that it is younger ones who have been laid off, affecting the company's age profile and with the result that attitudes towards older people have become unfavourable (Taylor 2006). The point here is that while governments are focused on long-term threats to social welfare systems and labour supply resulting from demographic change, older workers are facing a different and more immediate set of challenges. Popular policy and academic terms such as 'age management' and 'active ageing' may seem somewhat glib to managers facing the prospect of losing out to foreign competitors and to older workers contemplating uncertain futures.

Another lesson from the above case examples and from the evidence of Henkens et al. (2006) is that while business may currently be taking up the slack of older workers' employment, the picture could quickly change with a downturn in markets. Interest, where it exists, seems to be 'soft'. This complicated landscape is yet to be explored thoroughly, but it is clear that not all older workers will be able to take advantage of opportunities for working later. In fact, a more realistic scenario for some will be a transition to some form of early exit. This is rarely acknowledged nowadays amid the hyperbole of active ageing. Arguments for the prolongation of working life from advocates for older people hinging on the benefits accruing from active ageing fit neatly with the determination of many governments to role back welfare states and a 'welfare to work' ideology. Unfortunately, neglecting the realities of older workers' position in the labour market will result in a sub-class of older people trapped on an unemployment hinterland just as the early exit tide has turned. Their prospects are bleak. For those that follow them there are serious questions about the willingness or ability of policy-makers to do much to help. Some current commentators are not optimistic about older workers' prospects. For instance, Richard Sennett (2006) has referred to the 'spectre of uselessness' facing them as the jobs they were doing move to other countries. Although strongly reminiscent of the observations of many European commentators over more than a quarter of a century, Sennett's position does stand in stark contrast to many current views, for whom older workers' future is a bright one as populations age. How their labour market position would appear during a sudden economic downturn is a matter for speculation, although history and the evidence presented in this chapter should not give too much cause for optimism. European businesses trying to keep on competitive terms with foreign ones often see they have little choice but to remove older labour.

Conclusion

It is undeniably the case that the mass early retirement that featured so much in the 1980s and 1990s has ended, at least for now. Older workers, it is frequently argued, are on the brink of a new era of employment opportunities as the population of Europe ages and employers face a dwindling supply of labour. But are they really entering a 'golden age' of employment opportunities or is this a one-dimensional view that ignores the reality of modern labour markets? As demonstrated in this chapter, there is no particular reason to assume that older workers can look forward to such a future. Some, particularly those with high levels of skill, although not immune from the global forces acting on national labour markets, will continue to have a degree of choice over whether to work on or to retire. On the other hand, those with less relevant skills and those with disabilities or health problems that limit the kinds of work they can do will continue to face significant disadvantages. This familiar story seems to have been neglected in recent years. A naïve perspective on older workers' employment focuses solely on 'working later', while more thoughtful observers will consider the circumstances under which older workers will maintain links with the labour market, examining how population ageing will interact with the reorganization of industry as new markets open or markets decline, competition increases and alternative sources of labour supply emerge. The latter will also consider the destinations of older workers leaving full-time employment for flexible work and ask whether they are afforded equality of employment opportunity or can only access certain occupations or industrial sectors. Even if older workers' employment rates continue their generally upward trajectory, there will continue to be those who cannot maintain or achieve a foothold in the labour market and therefore have reduced prospects for a happy retirement. There will be a need for the continuation of the extensive work that has already mapped out the pathways to retirement (e.g. Kohli et al. 1991), but which updates it for the changing circumstances of globalizing labour markets. Current policies put much faith in the ability and willingness of the market to countenance ageing workforces and in instruments such as employment protection legislation, flexible retirement and lifelong learning to level the playing field for older workers. As demonstrated, the evidence for a strong positive employer response and for the effectiveness of such remedies is weak.

It is undoubtedly the case that some older workers with the right kinds of human capital will, if policy-makers have their way, soon be steering towards a bright future of labour market choices. By contrast, others will forever be trapped on the labour market event horizon, seemingly powerless to pull clear from an uncertain retirement, but with no alternative but to continue the struggle. The implication is that, however unfashionable a notion it would be in policy circles, it is carefully designed early retirement, not welfare to work, that will serve many older workers better into the foreseeable future.

References

Auer, P. and Fortuny, M. (2000) *Ageing of the Labour Force in OECD Countries: Economic and Social Consequences*. Geneva: International Labour Organization.

Frerichs, F. and Taylor, P. (2005) *Labour Market Policies for Older Workers and Demographic Change: A Comparative Analysis of Policy Approaches in Germany and the United Kingdom*. London: Anglo-German Foundation.

Guillemard, A-M. (1997) Re-writing social policy and changes within the life course organisation: a European perspective, *Canadian Journal on Aging*, 16(3): 441–64.

Guillemard, A–M. and Argoud, D. (2004) France: a country with a deep early exit culture, in T. Maltby, B. de Vroom, M-L Mirabile and E. Øverbye (eds) *Ageing and the Transition to Retirement: A Comparative Analysis of European Welfare States*, pp. 165–85. Aldershot: Ashgate.

Henkens, K., van Dalen, H. and Schippers, J. (2006) Managing an aging workforce: the role of employers, the Gerontological Society of America 59th Annual Scientific Meeting, Dallas, USA, 16–19 November.

Hotopp, U. (2005) The employment rate of older workers, *Labour Market Trends*, February, 73–88.

Kohli, M., Rein, M., Guillemard, A-M. and van Gunsteren, H. (eds) (1991) *Time for Retirement: Comparative Studies of Early Exit from the Labour Force*. Cambridge: Cambridge University Press.

Sennett, R. (2006) *The Culture of the New Capitalism*. London: Yale University Press.

Taylor, P. (2002) *New Policies for Older Workers*. Bristol: The Policy Press.

Taylor, P. (2006) *Employment Initiatives for an Ageing Workforce in the EU-15*. Luxembourg: Office for Official Publications of the European Communities.

5 Extensions to working lives in the information economy

Kerry Platman[1]

Introduction

The European Commission has set itself an ambitious goal of extending the working lives of its citizens. Mechanisms to raise employment rates and delay retirement among the older working population are part of a much broader, long-term strategy to become the most dynamic information economy in the world. By modernizing labour market structures under the Lisbon Strategy, it is said that Europe will be able to compete head-on with the newly industrialized giants of China, India and other low-cost emergent economies, as well as with advanced, innovation-driven economies such as the United States of America (USA) and Japan.

What are the difficulties facing member states in reconciling the need for suitable jobs for an ageing labour force with the need for competitive business practices to facilitate world-class European products and services? Is it possible to reconcile the need for flexibility in terms of organizational responses to rapidly changing global markets, with the need for welfare structures which deliver employment and retirement security? Authors such as Sennett (2006) suggest the forces of globalization will confine older workers to 'the spectre of uselessness' due to the rapid obsolescence of skills. Others have highlighted the enduring culture of early retirement which persists in many member states and the barriers which older workers face in securing the necessary training and career opportunities to sustain their working lives.

These issues are explored by focusing on the European findings of an international study of working practices and age-management approaches in the information technology (IT) sector. The sector is regarded as pivotal to a vibrant, knowledge-based economy, due to its rapid expansion in recent decades and the ongoing integration of advanced IT systems into established business processes. Yet the sector has also suffered a serious economic downturn and has an occupational profile which remains largely youthful, despite the maturing of the sector. What, then, are the prospects for extensions to working lives in the IT sector and, by implication, in other knowledge-intensive, globally competitive industries?

Extending our working lives

In response to predictions of a shrinking and ageing population, the European Union (EU) has agreed ambitious targets to improve labour participation rates for older workers by 2010. The Stockholm target, established at the 2001 European Council, set a goal for member states of increasing the average employment rate of older men and women (aged 55–64) to 50 per cent by 2010. The following year, the Barcelona target established a further aim of delaying by five years the average age at which older workers exited the labour market. These goals were seen as critical in the face of impending demographic change and predicted declines in the working-age population. Although the scale and timing of change will vary across member states, the total working-age population (15–64 years) of the EU is due to fall by 20.8 million between 2005 and 2030, creating unprecedented pressures on labour supply and welfare systems, and leading to forecasts of unsustainably low levels of economic growth (Commission of the European Communities 2005b).

The urgency of the task was restated more recently in a number of European Commission communications urging member states to develop strategies to suppress early retirement practices and lengthen the working lives of citizens (Commission of the European Communities 2005a, 2005b, 2005c, 2005d, 2006). Without more positive approaches to the ageing labour force, these documents warn of a Community which will fail to prosper against its global competitors. Its annual economic growth rate (measured in gross domestic product) is predicted to fall systematically from 2.4 per cent over the period 2004–2010 to 1.2 per cent between 2030 and 2050 (Commission of the European Communities 2006). Measures which specifically address the long-term effects of the decline in the working-age population (15–64 years) are part of a much broader attempt to position Europe as a dynamic and innovative global player, as detailed in the next section.

Devising a global strategy for Europe

Measures to extend and improve job opportunities for older (and younger) people across Europe are part of a wide-ranging strategic vision for Europe as a productive and world-leading global force. The Lisbon Strategy, revamped and clarified in 2005, lays out the mechanisms by which Europe will achieve its ambition to become 'the most competitive and dynamic knowledge-based economy in the world, capable of sustainable economic growth with more and better jobs and greater social cohesion' (European Council 2000, section I.5). European member states will need to remove the remaining internal barriers to trade and investment, while gaining improved access to external markets. They must recognize that knowledge and innovation are key drivers of productivity – 'the beating heart of European growth' (Commission of the European Communities 2005a) – and that world-class information technology and media sectors have long-term strategic value. At the same time, they should modernize labour market structures in order to end rigidities, improve labour mobility, facilitate transitions and invest in a highly skilled and adaptable workforce.

A strong theme to emerge from recent debates and policy documents at the European level is the promotion of flexibility alongside security (Schmid 1998, 2002; Wilthagen 2002). Keeping true to European values means supporting welfare structures, notably income support, employment protection and state pension provision, as well as achieving economic superiority in the global marketplace, in terms of high productivity, performance and growth (Commission of the European Communities 2005c). According to this perspective, Europe will undermine its core mission if, in its drive to compete (with the advanced, innovation-driven economies of the USA and Japan, and the emergent economies of China, India and other centres of low-cost labour), it fails to provide high-quality health care, satisfactory jobs for all, adequate state pensions and cohesion across the EU.

How far is it possible, though, to reconcile the goals of social justice in a rapidly ageing labour force with the need for aggressive, innovative and world-beating industrial players? On the one hand, this entails quality jobs for older workers, long-term investments in lifelong learning and employment rights offering protection against age discriminatory practices in the workplace. The quest for economic prosperity in a knowledge-based economy requires, on the other hand, competitive working practices, increasing use of 'atypical' contracts, high-risk innovation strategies, offshoring to emerging low-cost economies and inflows of highly skilled migrants. Rapidly changing economies require flexible labour markets which, in turn, result in rapid growth and renewal. This places ever greater burdens on workers and their employers to 'anticipate, trigger and absorb change' (Commission of the European Communities 2005a), to adapt to labour market shocks and to invest continually in new technologies and high-end skills. The risk is that competitive practices of the scale and intensity envisaged by the EU will result in poor-quality jobs, insecure forms of work and inadequate access to training and career opportunities for older generations of workers, especially those nearing retirement age.

Workforce ageing in the new economy

To examine these issues further, the chapter draws on the European findings of an international study of working practices in one sector at the forefront of the globally competitive knowledge economy: Information and Communication Technology (ICT). The sector is regarded as highly strategic in Europe for two main reasons. First, it has achieved above-average rates of growth and job creation over the last decade. ICT, covering both manufacturing and services, employed 6.7 million people in Europe (EU-25) in 2001, with an annual turnover of €1.6 billion (European Commission 2005). Second, the sector's innovations have the potential to permeate and improve cross-sector business processes and productivity. Although the 2000–1 downturn caused job losses and restructuring in many ICT enterprises, its annual turnover remains stronger than the more established European industries of car manufacturing and pharmaceuticals (Friedewald et al. 2004).

Yet, it has also been in the vanguard of offshoring practices, with a large number of IT programming and support functions being offshored to countries such as India and South Africa where labour costs are lower (Bradshaw et al. 2006). In addition, the age profile of the ICT workforce is highly skewed. Despite the maturing of the industry, it remains predominantly 'young' and male (Dixon 2002; Dixon and Addison 2000; Platman and Taylor 2004). The typical employment contract is permanent and full time, suggesting that opportunities for the kind of flexible extensions to working lives envisaged by policy-makers and pressure groups remain limited (see, for instance, Department for Work and Pensions 2006; Reday-Mulvey 2005).

The study focused on the employment relationship and working conditions in small- and medium-sized enterprises (SMEs), defined as employing between 5 and 249 staff (Forth et al. 2006). Such firms are seen as essential to the success of the Lisbon Strategy due to their role in fostering entrepreneurship, innovation and sustainable growth. They constitute 99 per cent of all enterprises in Europe and provide two-thirds of total employment (Commission of the European Communities 2005a: 16). Yet, in a tight labour market, they can struggle to compete for highly skilled labour against their larger rivals, undermining their capacity to grow and survive. Examining the ways in which SMEs navigate the financial and commercial risks of a global IT sector, against the backdrop of an ageing labour force, provides us with insights into the trade-off between business effectiveness on the one hand, and sustainable careers for workers on the other. The downturn in the IT sector in 2000–1, and the prolonged period of retrenchment which followed, provides an additional economic backdrop in which to view human resource management strategies in the sector.

The European findings reported here are part of a four-year international comparative study entitled *Workforce Ageing in the New Economy*, funded by the Social Sciences and Humanities Research Council of Canada. The study examined the histories of firms, their business processes and management practices, as well as the career trajectories of the people they employed. More details of the project are to be found at www.wane.ca. In Phase Two of the project, the international research team carried out a total of 55 case studies of SME firms specializing in IT software and services across the countries of Canada, the USA, Australia, the United Kingdom (UK), Netherlands and Germany. This chapter gives an overview of preliminary findings from the 15 SME case studies conducted in Europe: UK (7 SME cases), Netherlands (4) and Germany (4).

Methods

The European case studies were selected using a theoretical sampling approach, based on the work of Mason and others (Mason 1996; Finch and Mason 1990). The aim was to maximize variety among our case study group in order to reflect the diversity of the sector, in terms of niche markets, location, ownership, organizational structure, workforce composition, firm history and size. Nine of the fifteen European SMEs were operated by owner-managers, two were publicly listed, two were subsidiaries of larger companies, one was a cooperative and one was a non-profit enterprise. The median size of firms was 13 employees, with the largest employing 189 staff. Four of the firms were relatively long-established, having been formed between the late 1960s and early 1990s. Six of the firms had been operating since the late 1990s and a further five since 2001 or later. They were geographically spread, although the majority was located in high-tech corridors. The staff who worked for these firms were overwhelmingly male, reflecting the gender bias in the sector at the European and international level (Platman and Taylor 2004). Only one firm, a non-profit enterprise in the Netherlands, employed the same number of women as men. The remainder employed an average of 77 per cent men, slightly lower than the proportions to be found in the IT practitioner workforce as a whole in these three countries (Platman and Taylor 2004). The firms were also highly diverse in terms of the age profile of workers. Staff ranged in age from their early 20s to early 70s, although the vast majority were in their 30s and early 40s, reflecting the youthful age profile of the IT practitioner workforce as a whole (Comeau 2004).

It is important to say that these firms represent a survivor group, as do the IT practitioners they employed. The IT downturn after 2000 led to substantial job losses in the sector, and to many firms restructuring, merging or folding. The firms who took part in our study are those that survived this economic shock with sufficient optimism to feel they had a sufficiently sound future to take part in a relatively lengthy research project. In addition, the research teams required extensive access to the people and processes in each firm and this involved considerable time which a number of other firms we approached felt unable to give.

The fieldwork took place from November 2004 to September 2005 and involved face-to-face interviews with 105 individuals, observations of work processes, an online survey and corporate documents detailing the history of the firm. The interviews, a small number of which took place by telephone, involved semi-structured conversations with company owners, line managers and IT practitioners, including software designers, chief technology officers, customer support engineers, project managers and quality assurance consultants.

The next section gives a snapshot of key issues emerging from these case studies. Three aspects of day-to-day operations are highlighted, illustrating the intense pressures facing these firms. In a rapidly changing and volatile market environment, survival of the firm inevitably took priority over the individual needs and life stages of employees.

1 Customer responsiveness

These small- and mid-sized firms recognized that their survival and growth depended on their customer responsiveness and this presented smaller firms with particular difficulties in terms of staff capacity and internal resources. At certain times in an IT project's lifecycle, the pressures were especially intense. Firms often encountered unforeseen technical difficulties while developing their products or consultancy services. Equally, it was common for clients' needs to change midway through a project. Establishing a customer-facing presence – entailing delivery, speed and value for money – was a key driver of success among our case firms. This is illustrated by the way one of the UK firms had repositioned itself in an IT niche which was dominated by US rivals. The Chief Executive explained the success in terms of high visibility and rapid response:

> ... we've got a team of people out here now ... who are incredibly responsive in the marketplace ... If somebody, you know, if somebody approaches us ... then we respond initially very, very quickly,

> so that it creates the right sort of, uh, the right sort of uh appearance in the marketplace. And then subsequently ... we just start hitting the deadlines.

The formula had proved immensely successful. From near bankruptcy, the Chief Executive had orchestrated a management buyout of the firm and taken it to profitability within a space of less than two years. However, the pressures on staff had been substantial. The online survey data for this firm revealed high levels of stress, overall fatigue, anxiety and irritability. Memories of the near collapse of the firm were still fresh in the minds of many staff, leading them to work even harder in order to secure and expand the customer base and, in turn, improve their own job security. This was expressed by a woman employee in her late 20s who had been made redundant when the company was near to collapse but was later re-employed in her previous job. She was aware of the needs of the client and this had led to an intense and unrelenting work schedule. Justifying her willingness to accept this for the time being at least, she said: '... the reason I look at it is, just, I don't want to be redundant again. I don't want the company, I don't want to see the company go under again'.

Another example of customer responsiveness came from a highly innovative firm which was designing software systems for an international clientele. The firm had a branch in the USA which serviced its North American customers. The rest of the customer base, of around 1,000 clients, was supported by a team of four people and their manager at the firm's headquarters in the UK. The pressures facing the firm were summed up in the opening section of the interview with the manager, a woman in her mid-40s. Asked to give her title and describe her work, she replied:

> My title is International Support Manager. Which basically means that we look after all existing customers with valid maintenance contracts worldwide outside of North America and Canada. So our territories include South Africa, Australia, Asia Pacific. Just literally the whole world!

The pace of work was intense, but was particularly so during 'mission critical' phases where a slow response could undermine the operation of their products and, therefore, the functioning of IT systems on which their clients depended. She described the typical reaction of her firm, and its staff, during one of these phases:

> And it's all panic, panic and everybody's all hands to the pump, fix it, test it in QA [quality assurance]. And then we have the process of notifying resellers and third party vendors so they can amend their code in advance before we then go to the customers and say there's

> this problem you've got to upgrade your software or firmware. And this is every single customer ... So that's always extremely stressful.

Firms and their staff members who failed to perform sufficiently swiftly risked undermining the viability of operations, and thus the future success of the company. The need for timeliness in responding to customer needs presented a challenge for those individuals with caring responsibilities or who wished for a gradual exit out of the workforce. It appeared that the best form of job security these firms could deliver was a viable, long-term future. But this was directly related to the performance and response levels which staff could provide. Interviews with the oldest 'survivors' in these firms, those aged 45 years and over, revealed their willingness to remain highly adaptable to the constantly changing demands of their customers and to the increasingly complex task of delivering effective software solutions in a competitive market.

2 Cost constraints

The downturn in the IT sector after 2000 had affected the European firms in our study, more so for those offering general IT consultancy services than specialized software products. The downturn had gone hand in hand with a maturing IT sector and a more demanding and IT savvy clientele, leading to lower margins and tighter budgets. The effect of the recession had been so acute at one of the smallest of the case firms in the UK that the managing director negotiated a wage cut for staff in early 2002. Another firm had found it increasingly difficult to bid for IT projects due to the comparatively high cost base of his small UK firm compared to the much cheaper rates which those rivals with the capacity to offshore the majority of the work could offer. Although his firm could provide a better product and a more immediate personal service to UK clients, customers would often opt for the keenest price.

The margins had become so slender in the mid-sized German firm offering general consultancy services that staff were under pressure to cut any corners they could to save money. In the case of one of its most experienced and oldest consultants, this had led to an elaborate travel ritual in order to save money on airport and parking charges. The consultant would regularly take a far more complex, time-consuming and exhausting journey to visit one client in the extreme south of the country rather than use the more direct and more expensive route.

The operating costs, such as office rents, wage bills and fringe benefits, were under constant review by these firms. Many staff spoke of the need to take on multiple roles in order to cover the spread of expertise and responsibilities required by customers. Company owners and chief executives spoke of the importance of encouraging good teamworking and staff development, but this had to be achieved on the tightest of margins.

Many of the firms we studied had introduced imaginative devices to improve communication, commitment and loyalty among staff. But practices such as team-building weekends and evening socials could lead to a poor 'fit' between IT practitioners of different ages and cultural backgrounds. More critical were the inherent barriers to flexible schedules tailored to the worker and their life circumstances, rather than to the firm. Part-time working was seen as a risky exercise, due to the constant yet uncertain demands of the projects and tasks involved in software solutions. Part-time schedules for core IT work tended to be used in extreme cases and for limited periods, such as for women returning from maternity leave who were expected to resume full-time work at some point soon. The firms who had survived the IT downturn had done so by nurturing a high-commitment, high-delivery and high-staff-integration model of people management.

3 Rapidity of product development

Many of the staff involved in IT work in these case firms were relying on established programming languages and stable computing systems. However, there was recognition that mastery in such 'legacy' systems was not conducive to a long-term, sustainable career. Workers needed to keep abreast of the latest developments in their field and, unless they were fortunate enough to have such opportunities within their firm, they needed to do so in their own time.

The importance of this informal learning performed away from the office, out of regular working hours and in the privacy of the home, emerged strongly in the case of a number of software engineers in the innovative UK firm mentioned earlier. Their face-to-face interviews revealed the value they placed on this self-learning, in terms of career prospects, personal satisfaction and keeping abreast of the speed and breadth of technological advances. One senior software manager, who had turned a spare bedroom into an office-cum-'cave' of technological exploration, justified the hours he spent there in the following terms:

> I think an element of that is, I've always said to myself, I need to keep in touch, I need to keep up with technology. It's far harder to catch up if you fall behind. I believe that to keep up in the IT industry I have to invest some of my time outside of work doing that. If [UK company] doesn't pay me to keep up, for my own benefit and my future career, whatever happens in the future I need

> to keep up. And that's the best way of making myself employable, so that's my excuse for spending far too long in the office at home playing with computers.

Another of his colleagues, a project leader, pursued private client work on the side to keep abreast of emergent technologies. His comments reveal the dilemmas facing firms and their staff in pursuing untried but cutting-edge languages and platforms.

> One of the things that [UK COMPANY] does, which makes it a reasonably stable company, is we're based on very old, I say old, you know reasonably, tried and tested technologies ... So ... I get good experience and I keep my hand in ... I make myself much more employable and much more rounded by keeping up occasional contracts (with private clients).

Their learning took place in their spare time. Both had young children and wives who were the prime carers. They were free to use home time and holiday entitlements to pursue this out-of-office learning regime. They were pragmatic about the chances of their employer paying for training which could not be directly related to their current project. Customer pressures and project deadlines left little or no time for tangential learning.

The difficulties of offering the amount and type of learning which individuals felt they needed was illustrated by the case of a staff member wanting to take a project management training course in a programming language which his company did not use. This request had been refused, as the Chief Executive explained:

> ... it was a very personal request, a personal frolic that they wanted to do to enhance their own career at our expense, and they were naïve enough not to have recognised that we would have seen through that.

For the most part, individuals recognized that the way to keep abreast of technological change was to maintain a constant (private) interest. The recipe promoted by one Dutch IT worker was by constructing a portfolio of part-time roles and blurring the boundaries between work and home. He called it 'living the digital life', a system by which he would blend tasks, locations, hours and technologies to suit the demands of his employers and his family life. However, such methods demanded an intense and continuous commitment to the changing nature of tasks and technological innovations. IT practitioners appeared to be engaged in a system of bartering over access to learning: the more they engaged in upskilling at their own expense, the more they felt they could secure decent employment in the IT labour market. This, again, was conditional on individuals having the stamina, facilities and interest in such a trade-off.

The pressures of competitive global markets

A policy consensus has emerged over the need to extend working lives to sustain pension and welfare structures as the EU's labour force ages and shrinks in the coming decades. The difficulties in achieving this are substantial, however, as documented by a growing policy literature at the European and member state level (see, for example, Taylor 2006). Even in countries like the UK, where labour participation rates have grown among the 50+ age group since the mid-1990s, there is evidence that the obstacles to further increases in economic activity are substantial. Recent UK research has revealed the extent of chronic ill health among those people who have left the labour market ahead of state retirement age (Humphrey et al. 2003; Irving et al. 2005; Banks 2006). There is evidence of a complex interplay of factors leading to the premature exit of older workers. Two key drivers, in addition to health issues, are major 'shocks' such as redundancy, recession, industrial restructuring and organizational change, and care-giving for a spouse, grandchild(ren) and/or elderly relative, leading to an early exit from paid employment, or a move to a less demanding and lower-skilled job.

Less well understood is the impact of global labour supplies and competitive global industries on the opportunities to extend working lives in Europe. As Estes et al. (2003) note, we need a clearer understanding of the pressures facing older people as a consequence of accelerating global change. Globalized markets are transforming the location, speed and intensity of work flows and the means of communicating with customers. The integration and widespread take-up of ICT has led to an intensification of competition by collapsing geographical distances and time zones. There is an increasing degree of interdependency and interconnectedness between regional, national and international economies and enterprises. The technology which allows European enterprises to reach new markets beyond the Eurozone is also the same technology which provides access to our own markets, threatening the stability of established players and the viability of start-ups. A favoured approach in Europe is to encourage the development of high-end goods and services by relying on knowledge, creativity and innovation. Such capacities become 'the key differentiating factor in competitiveness' (Wilson et al. 2006: 25), placing heavy burdens on individuals to maintain these high-level skills, creative energies and innovative capacities.

Is it possible, then, to reconcile these dual aims, of world-beating competitiveness on the one hand and high employment participation for an ageing labour force on the other? Two complementary theoretical approaches suggest this is an ambition worth striving for. The concepts of flexicurity and transitional labour markets have evolved as separate although overlapping approaches to the challenges of modernization and renewal facing EU countries. The 'flexibility-security nexus', as Wilthagen (2002) calls it, advocates a balancing act, or trade-off, between the needs of European citizens, the business pressures facing employers and the ability of regulatory and legislative frameworks to effect change. Likewise, Schmid argues that transitory employment states are an important labour market dynamic underpinning global economies (Schmid 1998; Schmid 2002). They are a consequence of, if not a precondition for, economies based on technological innovation and international competition. However, one of the most risk-saturated of these is the transition from permanent employment to retirement, and such transitions are exacerbated in sectors dependent on ICT since they tend to devalue traditional skills in a far more radical way than the more traditional skillsets learned in mechanics and engineering. Schmid and Schömann (2004, see chapter X) suggest, somewhat controversially, that older workers may be better placed in other kinds of jobs, away from the rapidly evolving IT-driven sectors and occupations. They offer sectors such as retailing, care work, financial advice and counselling as potentially more viable alternatives. However, this raises the spectre of an age-segmented approach to labour force participation in an ageing society, and one which could exacerbate skills supply and labour retention issues in certain occupations and industries.

The findings of the *Workforce Ageing in the New Economy* study highlight the relentless business pressures facing small- and medium-sized enterprises operating in global, high-tech markets. It is important to acknowledge that the findings relate to firms employing fewer than 250 staff. It is possible that the fortunes of older IT professionals in the public sector, or in larger firms, might be different although the scale of restructuring which followed the IT downturn after 2000, coupled with trends in offshoring among the larger employers of IT staff, suggests this is unlikely to be the case. Further research is needed to test this.

An important and perhaps inevitable feature of highly competitive, high-tech markets is a set of business and employment practices to match. The three earlier sections go some way towards detailing the dimensions of this reality. The survival of these firms was dependent on them offering responsive services tailored to their potential, new and existing customers. But these services and products also had to be delivered at the right price, in competition with rivals who could undercut costs by a substantial margin. At the same time, emergent technologies were creating new opportunities, but also new threats, to the niche markets in which these firms operated, and to the long-term career prospects of their IT professionals.

A number of recent reports published by the European Foundation for the Improvement in Working Lives have stressed the need to build greater working-time flexibility over the life course, and permit a more individualized approach to work-endings (Naegele et al. 2003; Anxo et al. 2005; Klammer and Keuzenkamp 2005). Yet, in line with findings of an earlier study on ageing among media professionals (Platman 2004), the results reported here suggest that any attempt to engineer a gradual transition into retirement risks difficulties, due to the need for firms to offer instant, cutting-edge services in a highly competitive marketplace.

Small- and mid-sized firms who are competing in high-tech, global industries are faced with formidable pressures in order to deliver profitable services and products. There are limits to how much flexibility and security a firm can offer in a climate of fluctuating demand, fierce cost competition and uncertain technological progression. The firms involved in our *Workforce Ageing in the New Economy* study had survived the IT recession but, in many instances, the immediate future remained uncertain. The best these firms could offer their staff was a stimulating working environment in which there were prospects of future growth. These were demand-driven, problem-focused enterprises. Developing systems or procedures which were designed to retain staff for longer, and beyond retirement age, was well down the list of priorities if the business was to survive amid such fierce competition.

Notes

1 The author would like to thank the European project team involved in the *Workforce Ageing in the New Economy* study: Philip Taylor, WANE Europe team leader; Di Hinds and Sue Tostevin, University of Cambridge, UK; Katalin Velladics and Kène Henkens, Netherlands Interdisciplinary Demographic Institute; and Corinna Barkholdt and Frerich Frerichs, University of Dortmund, Germany. This project was funded by the Social Sciences and Humanities Research Council of Canada (SSHRCC) and led by Dr Julie McMullin, Associate Professor in the Department of Sociology at the University of Western Ontario, Canada. Finally, thanks are due to the firms and their staff who gave so generously of their time to take part in the research.

References

Anxo, D., Boulin, J.Y., Fagan, C., Cebrian, I., Keuzenkamp, S., Klammer, U., Klenner, C., Moreno, G. and Toharia, L. (2005) *Working Time Options over the Life Course: New Work Patterns and Company Strategies*. Dublin: European Foundation for the Improvement of Living and Working Conditions.

Banks, J. (2006) Economic capabilities, choices and outcomes at older ages, *Fiscal Studies*, 27 (3), 281–311.

Bradshaw, D., Brice, H., Codling, P., Hanaghan, K., Hayward, D., Holway, R. and Masood, S. (2006) *The Impact of Global Sourcing on the UK Software and IT Services Sector*, Ovum/Department of Trade & Industry (www.dti.gov.uk/files/file32496.pdf).

Comeau, T.D. (2004) *Cross-national Comparison of Information Technology Employment,* WANE International Report No. 5, University of Western Ontario.

Commission of the European Communities (2005a) *Communication to the Spring European Council: Working Together for Growth and Jobs.* Brussels: Commission of the European Communities.

Commission of the European Communities (2005b) *Confronting Demographic Change: A New Solidarity Between the Generations, Green Paper.* Brussels: Commission of the European Communities.

Commission of the European Communities (2005c) *European Values in a Globalised World.* Brussels: Commission of the European Communities.

Commission of the European Communities (2005d) *Lisbon Action Plan Incorporating EU Lisbon Programme and Recommendations for Actions to Member States for Inclusion in their National Lisbon Programmes, Companion document.* Brussels: Commission of the European Communities.

Commission of the European Communities (2006) *The Demographic Future of Europe: From Challenge to Opportunity.* Brussels: Commission of the European Communities.

Department for Work and Pensions (2006) *Security in Retirement: Towards a New Pensions System, White Paper.* Norwich: The Stationery Office.

Dixon, M. (2002) *Information Technology Practitioner Skills in Europe.* Frankfurt: CEPIS (Council of European Professional Informatics Societies).

Dixon, M. and Addison, L. (2000) *Analysis of the Information Technology Labour Market.* London: Information Technology National Training Organisation.

Estes, C.L., Biggs, S. and Phillipson, C. (2003) *Social Theory, Social Policy and Ageing: A Critical Introduction.* Maidenhead: Open University Press.

European Commission (2005) *Key Indicators on the Competitiveness of EU's ICT Industry.* Brussels: Enterprise and Industry Directorate-General.

European Council (2000) *Presidency Conclusions of the Lisbon European Council,* European Council (www.ue.eu.int/ueDocs/cms_Data/docs/pressData/en/ec/00100-r1.en0.htm).

Finch, J. and Mason, J. (1990) Decision-taking in the fieldwork process: theoretical sampling and collaborative working, in R.G. Burgess (ed.) *Studies in Qualitative Methodology*, pp. 25–50. London: JAI Press.

Forth, J., Bewley, H. and Bryson, A. (2006) *Small and Medium-sized Enterprises: Findings from the 2004 Workplace Employment Relations Survey*, ESRC, ACAS, PSI, NIESR and DTI.

Friedewald, M., Kimpeler, S., Hawkins, R., Poel, M., Lengrand, L., Chatrie, I. and Rachidy, J. (2004) *Benchmarking National and Regional Policies in Support of the Competitiveness of the ICT Sector in the EU. Final Report*. Brussels: European Commission.

Humphrey, A., Costigan, P., Pickering, K., Stratford, N. and Barnes, M. (2003) *Factors Affecting the Labour Market Participation of Older Workers*. Leeds: Corporate Document Services.

Irving, P., Steels, J. and Hall, N. (2005) *Factors Affecting the Labour Market Participation of Older Workers: Qualitative Research*. Leeds: Corporate Document Services.

Klammer, U. and Keuzenkamp, S. (2005) *Working Time Options Over the Life Course: Changing Social Security Structures*. Dublin: European Foundation for the Improvement of Living and Working Conditions.

Mason, J. (1996) *Qualitative Researching*. London: Sage Publications.

Naegele, G., Barkholdt, C., de Vroom, B., Goul Andersen, J. and Kramer, K. (2003) *A New Organisation of Time Over Working Life*. Dublin: European Foundation for the Improvement of Living and Working Conditions.

Platman, K. (2004) 'Portfolio careers' and the search for flexibility in later life, *Work, Employment & Society*, 18(3): 573–99.

Platman, K. and Taylor, P. (2004) *Workforce Ageing in the New Economy: A Comparative Study of Information Technology Employment*, University of Cambridge (www.wane.ca/otherpubs.htm).

Reday-Mulvey, G. (2005) *Working Beyond 60: Key Policies and Practices in Europe*. Basingstoke: Palgrave Macmillan.

Schmid, G. (1998) Transitional labour markets: a new European employment strategy, *Discussion Paper FS I 98–206*, Wissenschaftszentrum Berlin für Sozialforschung, Berlin.

Schmid, G. (2002) Transitional labour markets and the European social model: towards a new employment compact, in G. Schmid and B. Gazier (eds) *The Dynamics of Full Employment: Social Integration Through Transitional Labour Markets*, pp. 393–435. Cheltenham: Edward Elgar.

Schmid, G. and Schömann, K. (2004) *Managing Social Risks Through Transitional Labour Markets: Towards a European Social Model*. Amsterdam: SISWO/ Institute for the Social Sciences (www.siswo.uva.nl/tlm/root_files/ seminalpaper).

Sennett, R. (2006) *The Culture of the New Capitalism*. London: Yale University Press.

Taylor, P. (2006) *Employment Initiatives for an Ageing Workforce in the EU15*. Dublin: European Foundation for the Improvement of Living and Working Conditions.

Wilson, R., Homenidou, K. and Dickerson, A. (2006) *Working Futures 2004–2014: National Report*. Wath-upon-Dearne: Sector Skills Development Agency.

Wilthagen, T. (2002) The flexibility-security nexus: new approaches to regulating employment and labour markets, *British Journal of Industrial Relations Conference*, Cumberland Lodge, The Great Park, Windsor, September 16–17.

6 Older workers in social care: undervalued and overlooked?

Jill Manthorpe and Jo Moriarty

> I still have lots to offer. I'm very happy in my work and it's very rewarding. I'm not ready to lie down yet!
>
> (Social Services Officer, Bridgend County Borough Council, Wales, Age Positive 2007)

It is a paradox that while social care is predominantly concerned with the support of older people, the ageing of the social care workforce is generally ignored. To some extent, this reflects the marginalization of social care in debates about employment and work. It also reflects the complexities of the area across Europe where social care is generally loosely defined and its boundaries with the health care sector and with family care are blurred. This chapter looks at the shape of the social care sector and its workforce to outline the current challenges and trends, to consider issues arising for older workers who are professionally qualified and those who are not, and it illustrates some activities in the sector by drawing on organizational and personal case stories. While most social care is provided by family and friends, this chapter considers paid employment. There is much to learn from this sector since is it female dominated, has great diversity and is one of the main sectors where migrant workers have often found employment. Furthermore, talking about older social care workers in any part of Europe raises issues about globalization and ageing.

Defining social care

The term 'social care' is not commonly used outside England and has only a limited history in this country. Nonetheless, as an umbrella term it has its uses since it focuses attention on part of Europe's workforce that is often subsumed under health-related discussions, and marginalized as work that is temporary or only a small part of a family's income. In the United Kingdom (UK) it has been generally used to provide a generic label for the staff who worked in residential care homes and other social services who are not professionally qualified social workers, rather than to describe the work or role that is undertaken (Platt 2007). The Commission for Social Care Inspection (CSCI) defines social care as:

> Cover[ing] a wide range of services, which are provided by local authorities and the independent sector. Social care comes in many forms, such as care at home, in day centres or by way of residential or nursing homes. The term also covers services such as providing meals on wheels to the elderly, home help for people with disabilities and fostering services.
>
> (CSCI, undated)

In Scotland, the term 'social work services' is used more often than social care and in Northern Ireland the equivalent is 'personal social services'. Social care work spans several occupations. These include:

- social care staff including professional staff: social workers, care assistants, and so on;
- health professionals and staff employed in the social care sectors (allied health professionals nurses, health care assistants;
- ancillary staff (cleaners, catering staff, porters, etc.)
- managers (for various levels, context and roles);
- administration and clerical.

(Wanless 2006: 124)

Social care work in Europe

Social care work has been an important source of job growth in the European Union (EU) in recent years. Between 1980 and 1996 service sector employment in the EU increased by around 19 million with the largest area of growth occurring in the 'care' services' (health, social services, education), various business services and environmental activities (Anxo and Fagan 2001: 94). Despite this, much more attention has been given to the organization and provision of services than to the care workforce (Ewijk et al. 2002; Cameron and Moss 2007). This study remains our major source of information on the social care workforce in Europe. It was undertaken across six EU countries (Spain, Hungary, the Netherlands, the UK, Denmark and Sweden) and showed that the workforce is divided into two tiers; the larger workforce involved in providing direct care who are mainly untrained or have vocational qualifications, and a smaller workforce consisting of those employed in professional occupations, such as social work. Table 6.1 shows the proportions of people employed in social care in the four countries for which comparable data was available (Ewijk et al. 2002). The 'social work associate professionals' category includes youth workers and community workers as well as social workers.

The research also revealed that most people employed in care work in Demark are working full time but those in the Netherlands and the UK were typically working part time. This means that comparing the social care workforce across Europe is not easy but nonetheless there are commonalities. One of these, as this chapter demonstrates, is the ageing of Europe's social care workforce. Responses to this challenge, however, are varied and much depends on the local context.

Table 6.1 Proportion of the total workforce employed in social care (percentage)

Occupational group	Denmark	Spain	Sweden	UK
Personal care	7.4	2.2	10.5	4.2
Social work associate professionals	0.5	0.2	0.8	1.0

Source: Ewijk et al. (2002), adapted from Table 7.1, p. 69.

Social care work in the UK

The social care sector in the UK is a complex set of sub-sectors, with key differences in terms of activity, the labour market and the skills context. The sector comprises three main sub-sectors – care or support for older people, other disabled people with physical or mental health problems, including learning disabilities, and children. Social care for older people is the largest in terms of employers and employees; followed by support for adults with learning disabilities (intellectual impairment); then support for adults with physical disabilities; while social care for children in the care of local authorities is the smallest sector. There are about 25,000 employers in the care sector in England (Eborall 2003). Most are private and voluntary organizations, ranging in size from companies with thousands of employees, to small family businesses. Within care homes as many as 95 per cent of staff are female; on average they are aged around 40 years, and most work part time, around 25 hours per week. Labour turnover in the sector is high, with some care homes estimating it to be as much as 30 per cent. Average job tenure in a particular home is about three years (Machin and Manning 2002).

The statutory or public sector, Local Authorities (LAs) and their Social Services Departments (currently now known as adult services departments), are responsible for the commissioning of independent (private and voluntary sector) providers to provide services in care home and through home care agencies. They also provide a range of services, including assessment and care management, generally done by social workers. Social care services for children are the smallest in terms of the number of children being supported and the size of homes (Gospel and Thompson 2003) with an estimated 55,000 children in care of various kinds and about 1,000 children's homes in England.

Numbers

Although differences in the way that the social care workforce is categorized across Europe are to be expected, it is even difficult to estimate the size of the total UK social care workforce because of differences in the way that information is categorized and recorded across all four countries. The most recent published estimates suggest that the 'traditional', or 'core', social care workforce in England numbers 922,000 people, increasing to 1,598,000 if occupations such as foster carers for children are included serving a population of 50,762,900 people (Office for National Statistics 2007). In Scotland, the workforce is thought to number 138,000 people (Scottish Executive 2006b) and the population is 5,116,900 (Office for National Statistics 2007) and in Wales, with a population of 2,965,900, the size of the social care workforce, including child care, learning and development is estimated to be 88,773 (Care Council for Wales undated). The Northern Ireland social care workforce is thought to number 40,140 people (Department of Health Social Services and Public Safety 2006), serving a population of 1,741,600. Based on these estimates, and without taking any account of the levels of disability or need within the population, this suggests that the social care workforce is proportionally larger in Wales than in the rest of the UK.

Demographics

Age

Like its counterpart in health services (see Chapter 11), the social care workforce is often described as an 'ageing workforce' (McNair and Flynn 2006). Over 60 per cent of social care workers are estimated to be aged 35 years and over (Skills for Care 2007a). Figure 6.1 shows the age distribution of staff employed by local authorities in England (Local Authority Workforce Intelligence Group 2006). It highlights how the majority of social care staff is aged 40 years and over and in some occupations, particularly home care, the proportions are even higher.

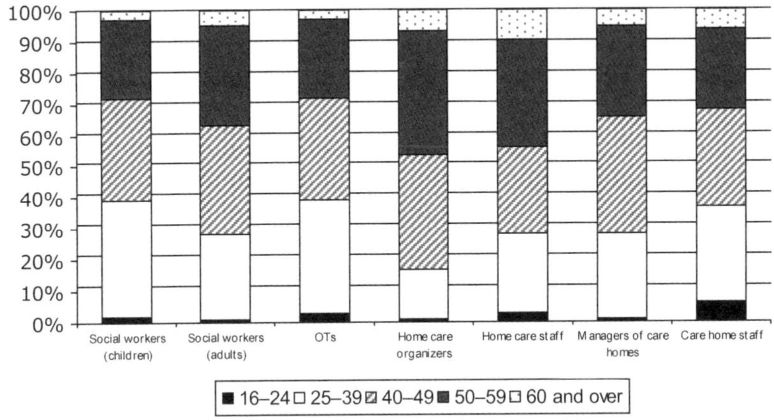

Source: Local Authority Workforce Intelligence Group (2006), adapted from Table 4.

This picture is not atypical. As Table 6.2 shows, in their study Ewijk and colleagues (2002) found a similar concentration of older workers in the social care workforce in mainland Europe, with strikingly few people younger than 25 years working in the sector.

Table 6.2 Age distribution of social care employees and total employed population

Occupational group	Denmark	Spain	Sweden	UK
Personal care				
15–24	16	15	10	11
25–44	50	56	51	51
45+	34	29	39	37
Social work associate professionals				
15–24	4	17	12	6
25–44	53	72	51	55
45+	43	12	38	38
All employed people				
15–24	15	13	9	14
25–44	49	55	49	52
45+	37	33	44	35

Source: Ewijk et al. (2002), adapted from Table 7.3, p. 72.

However, in the UK there are some age differences within work settings. The childcare workforce tends to be younger than the adult workforce; for example, staff working in children's nurseries have an average age of 24 (Cameron et al. 2002).

Gender

The gendered nature of care work is well known (Balloch et al. 1999; Ungerson 2000). The tendency for women to be in different jobs or occupations to those of men is known as horizontal segregation. Social care provides a striking example of this in that there are, on average, four women workers for every one man. This ratio is consistent across the UK (Department of Health Social Services and Public Safety 2006; Scottish Executive 2006b; Care Council for Wales undated) and a similar pattern emerges across the rest of Europe so that, even in countries such as Spain where women's participation in the labour force is much lower than that of men, almost 90 per cent of direct care workers are women (Ewijk et al. 2002).

However, the relationship between care work and gender is nuanced (Ewijk et al. 2002). The proportion of men found in the sector varies across different occupations and settings. For example, Gospel and Thompson (2003) found higher proportions of men working in group homes for people with learning disabilities whereas in other areas, such as childminding or nursery nursing, the proportion of men is even lower than across the sector as a whole (Cameron et al. 1999; Rolfe et al. 2003). Furthermore, the social care workforce also provides an example of vertical segregation whereby, within a particular occupation, women tend to hold the lower status and lower rewarded positions. Thus, while women are estimated to constitute around 84 per cent of the workforce, they make up only 67 per cent of senior managers (Skills for Care 2007a).

Explanations for these gender differences are complex and are attributable to a number of factors. These include stereotyped ideas about what constitutes so-called 'women's work' (Christie 1998; McLean 2003; Christie 2006), structural influences upon career progression including the higher proportion of men with professional qualifications, the higher proportions of women working part time and/or who have taken a career break (Davey et al. 2000; Davey 2002), and other less tangible ways in which men may continue to be advantaged in occupations in which women predominate, such as being more likely to affirm the professional nature and quality of their performance at work or being more conscious of the need to 'stand out' in the competition (Cross and Bagilhole 2002; Lupton 2006).

The gendered nature of social care also raises a further paradox that, although the workforce as a whole has an older age profile and care providers report many staff vacancies, it does not seem to have provided an attractive route to employment for economically inactive older men who may previously have worked in heavy industry (Esping-Andersen 1999). In the UK population as a whole, working-age men and women have different patterns of economic activity at most ages and it is striking that in the five years immediately preceding state pension 44 per cent of men aged 60–64 are economically inactive compared with 36 per cent of women aged 55–59 (Office for National Statistics 2006: 42). While this is an under-researched area, it may be that the reluctance of many older men to become involved in social organizations or services providing social support, either as volunteers or members (Davidson et al. 2003) might discourage them from working in communal social care settings.

Ethnicity

Like nursing (Beishon et al. 1995), social care in the UK has always attracted a comparatively high proportion of staff from minority ethnic groups (Butt et al. 1991; Balloch et al. 1999). Eight per cent of the total UK population is from a minority ethnic group (Office for National Statistics 2002), a similar proportion to that found in the social care workforce (Ewijk et al. 2002). Given the age structure of the population from a minority ethnic group with higher numbers of children aged 0–16 and the employment gaps that exist between the numbers of people from minority ethnic groups in paid employment (Clark and Drinkwater 2007), this suggests that social care represents an important area of work for people from minority ethnic groups. While many have been attracted to this area of employment because they find it interesting and rewarding, it is also known that people from black and minority ethnic groups are over-represented in occupations with low pay in the UK (Clark and Drinkwater 2007; Low Pay Commission 2007), such as care work. For example, 40 per cent of the social care workforce in London is from a minority ethnic group (Robinson and Banks 2005), although people from minority ethnic groups constitute 29 per cent of the local population overall (Owen 2001). Indeed, even within the sector, there have been some suggestions that people from minority ethnic groups are over-represented among those employed on a temporary (or contingency) basis in social care (Conley 2003) with worse terms and conditions of employment than their counterparts on permanent contracts, meaning that, in some settings, social care is an ethnically segmented occupation, in addition to being gender-segregated.

Given the numbers of people from minority ethnic groups in their 50s and 60s who have worked in social care in the UK, our knowledge about them is surprisingly scant. This is mainly because of the failure of published information on the workforce to disaggregate information about ethnicity and age. However, evidence from a study of older people from minority ethnic groups which included some interviews with people working in social care (Barnes and Taylor 2006) suggested that many faced particular issues that had implications for the degree of choice they had about working in later life, including the impact of lifelong low earnings on savings and pension income in retirement, the lower frequency of dual income households, and the need to send remittances to their country of origin. Disentangling the combined influences of discrimination on the grounds of age, gender and ethnicity experienced by older workers remains methodologically challenging. Social care would be an excellent exemplar for any such study.

The extent to which the UK picture mirrors that across Europe as a whole cannot be estimated because of differences in the way that ethnicity is recorded (Ewijk et al. 2002). However, there is increasing evidence that care work is increasingly associated with migration in Europe, partly due to the 'feminization of migration' in terms of the numbers of women leaving their countries of birth and partly due to the strategies that migrating women adopt in order to find employment where there are growing numbers of older people and where their access to other parts of the labour market may be restricted (Hillmann 2005). This phenomenon is particularly apparent in Italy where comparatively low public provision and demographic profile of the population (below replacement fertility levels) have led to informal employment of many non-Italian-born workers, known as *badanti* (attendant), as domestic carers. Palese et al.'s (2004) study of a group of *badanti* working in the Friuli Venezia Giulia region revealed a female workforce whose average age was 50 (ranging from 26 to 72 years) and who were often working in roles for which they might be perceived as overeducated. Most of the women had decided to work abroad for economic reasons either because their incomes and pensions at home were insufficient to support their families or because work was not available. Recruitment was either through private agencies or personal contact. Work conditions varied and many experienced feelings of isolation and loneliness, as well as the physical impacts of often extensive and demanding care responsibilities. Palese et al. (2004) anticipated that the *badanti* were becoming an increasing important component of the social care workforce in Italy and it is possible that the expansion of other cash for care or consumer-directed support might lead to similar developments in other European states.

Earnings and pensions

In England the costs of labour make up around half the costs of providing home care and between half and two-thirds of the costs in care homes (Wanless 2006: xv). This means that the average level of earnings received by those working in social care has become an important consideration for funders and the public purse because the way in which social care is purchased and provided is so price-sensitive (Knapp et al. 2001; Forder et al. 2004). Social care workers were one of the groups to benefit most from the introduction of the national minimum wage in 1999 in that, at the time, their wages were among the lowest in the UK (Machin and Manning 2002) and social care employers were one of the groups most concerned about the impact of this legislation (Grimshaw 2002; Grimshaw and Carroll 2006). Currently, data from the Annual Survey of Hours and Earnings (Office for National Statistics undated) shows that the average hourly rate of a care worker in the UK is currently just over £7 while a social worker might expect to earn £14 and a community worker or other associate professional would receive £11. However, wages in the private sector (where most care workers are employed) tend to be lower (Low Pay Commission 2007: xv). Furthermore, while the introduction of the national minimum wage has raised the pay of many care workers, in doing so it has caused significant wage compression at the bottom end of the wage distribution, meaning that many care workers still do not get the opportunity to earn higher wages and thus decent pensions through experience, skill acquisition or seniority (Machin et al. 2002).

Although Table 6.3 uses data collected before the introduction of the minimum wage in 1999, and is thus consequently now rather old, it remains valuable because it uses purchasing power parities, which eliminate price differentials between countries and so permit comparisons to be made. The table reveals two important messages. The first is that in all four countries, care workers earn less than the average person in full-time employment. The second is that while social welfare associate professionals in Denmark, the UK and Sweden earned broadly similar amounts, this was not true of care workers. Strikingly, only in Denmark, and to a lesser extent Sweden, could their earnings be seen as broadly comparable with average earnings as whole.

Table 6.3 Annual earnings of full- and part-time social care workers, 1995

	Denmark		**Spain**		**Sweden**		**UK**	
	PT	FT	PT	FT	PT	FT	PT	FT
Personal care	19,466	23,364	6,417	14,370	11,887	17,513	3,668	14,557
Social work associate professionals	23,992	29,350	8,181	28,016	13,001	21,590	7,164	27,094
Total in employment	18,099	25,069	6,725	19,841	10,746	19,895	5,348	21,592

Source: Ewijk et al. (2002), adapted from Table 8.3, p. 82.

This situation is largely attributable to factors identified above: the historical undervaluing of women's work (Grimshaw and Rubery 2007) and to the high degree of occupational segregation and part-time employment; two factors that contribute significantly to the gender pay gap (Anderson et al. 2001). The gender pay gap in the UK is currently 12.6 per cent between men and women in full-time paid employment but 40 per cent among those in part-time paid employment (Government Equalities Office 2008). As many as 50 per cent of the social care workforce is in part-time paid employment (Eborall 2005) and so women too suffer a pensions gap in later life if they have been employed in the social care sector.

Union membership is very low in the sector, with the exception of Local Authority care homes and social work, thus reducing individual workers' ability to challenge age or other discriminations. Indeed, Machin and Manning (2002) found that non-professional staff in social care often have weak or no employment contracts and even within the public sector, these contracts may lead to difficulties in planning income since 'zero hours' contracts mean there are few guarantees over employment or pay. For example, Francis and Netten (2003) found that two-thirds of one local authority's home care workers were on such contracts.

The composition of the social care workforce continues to be dominated by women seeking part-time paid employment and concerns have long been expressed about how this influences both the status and levels of remuneration that social care work attracts (Ungerson 2000; Eyers and Bryan 2006; Wanless 2006). The contracting out or outsourcing of services to the independent sector has also led to increasing fragmentation in terms of the number of employers. Taken together, this has made it harder to undertake the sorts of analysis aimed at establishing causal relationships, such as the impact of motivation upon retention or the factors that lead to early retirement or indeed to continuation after retirement in the social care sector. Workforce planning in this sector continues to be comparatively unsophisticated and there has only been a limited amount of work modelling projections of future supply and demand (e.g. Hancock et al. 2007).

Recruitment and retention

On the face of it, the social care sector might be a rich source of employment for older workers. The vacancy rate is double that for all types of industrial, commercial and public employment (Department of Health/Department for Education and Skills 2006) and the Commission for Social Care Inspection (CSCI) (2006) describes it as an area with 'chronic difficulties' in staffing. The interest in employing or retaining older workers is rising but not high profile, with some exceptions reported below. Parallel debates took place in the

United States of America (USA) some years previously, and we know more about the sector's views of older workers and older people's views of the social care sector from this source (Hwalek and Essenmacher 2005). Data from the US Operation (meaning for Older Workers: Ready, Willing and ABLE) ABLE projects reveal that:

- people aged 55 years (mature) and over are interested in paraprofessional health work (social care);
- employers have positive perceptions of mature workers;
- real and perceived deterrents to hiring mature workers include perceptions that this would entail greater health benefits expenditure by employers; that age discrimination laws mean that older workers cannot be targeted for recruitment; that older workers have to rely on public transport to get to work; that older workers are unwilling to use technology; that their training will incur costs; and that their wage expectations are high;
- home care work may be more appealing to older workers than care home work;
- new avenues for recruitment may reach older people better (e.g. advertising in senior centres, work and training organizations and places of worship);
- mature workers may be particularly interested in jobs that are relationship-centred and these may not be plentiful;
- stereotypes about physical capacity problems in later life exist and may be too generalized;
- employment and training organizations can overcome possible limits in information technology knowledge and skills.

(Kosniewski and Hwalek 2006)

Other work has identified examples where older workers are seen as offering advantages in terms of life experience and flexibility.

Box 6.1 Reintegrating older workers into employment

Passantenhuis Day Centre

The Passantenhuis Day Centre in Belgium provides care for older people and has a policy of trying to employ people aged over 45 as they have 'more experience of life'. This service works under the Flemish government 'back to work' scheme, targeted at unskilled workers who have been unemployed for over a year. Staff are trained, stay for one year, and the Centre provides an opportunity for them to be reintegrated into the labour market. Training is provided by the back to work scheme, but this is reported to be 'not extensive' and to be of 'low skills'.

L'Incontro Cooperative (Italy)

This small not-for-profit organization manages two residential homes for older people and an occupational day centre for younger adults in the Treviso region of Italy. The Cooperative relies mainly on older workers who have taken early retirement. As well as the social care activities mentioned above, the Cooperative also runs an employment service. Older workers are offered part-time work and job-sharing opportunities. This is regarded as offering them flexibility but also makes the service cost effective. The Cooperative considers that this employment practice leads to better quality care as the work is difficult and so shorter working hours mean that staff are not so stressed. As a result of offering flexible working hours to all employees, absenteeism is reduced. Turnover is also reported to be lower.

Source: Walker (1997).

In the voluntary and private sectors, vacancy rates seem to be lower than in the statutory sector but the turnover rate appears to be higher (Skills for Care 2007b). Overall, vacancies appear to be higher in care homes and among children's social work teams (Eborall 2005; Local Authority Workforce Intelligence Group 2006). However, many of the vacancies in social care are termed as 'hard to fill' and these are generally attributed to the existence of skills gaps (i.e. there is a shortage of suitably qualified candidates), rather than to there being an overall shortage of applicants (Learning and Skills Council 2006). This may be encouraging for older staff who may possess skills and experience that are in short supply and may account for some of the initiatives reported in Box 6.2 by Age Positive (undated) and Bennett et al. (2007).

Box 6.2 Flexible employment patterns

Wokingham District Council in the south-east of England aims to recruit retiring social care workers, particularly for sessional and casework. It offers training to older workers, and disseminates this to encourage others. Local mature students on social care courses are targeted for recruitment. Carers' leave is available and for those who have been out of care work for some time, a Return to Care campaign offers refreshment training and encouragement.

(Age Positive undated)

The Camden and Islington Mental Health and Social Care Trust

This Social Care Trust is a combination of NHS and local authority social care services in Inner London. The Trust has a *Valuing Diversity* policy that covers age, gender, religion, sexuality, disability and part-time or fixed-term employees. In addition, it has a Workforce Age Action Plan that promotes flexible working options and flexible retirement options and is exploring being an Age Positive Champion. The Trust offers options to Wind Down and to Step Down that enable staff to preserve pension rights earned at a higher level if they work in other areas. Others take up the option of retiring and coming back part time or work in winter peak times. The Trust treats requests for flexibility in the context of patient and team needs, but there is a right of appeal if a member of staff is unhappy with decisions. Staff have six days entitlement for paid special leave; for example, for emergences around caregiving responsibilities, and they can take 6–12 months unpaid leave for caregiving, as well as temporary reductions in hours or career breaks of up to five years.

(Bennett et al. 2007)

In terms of turnover, there is evidence that most social care workers leave to work for another social care employer or the NHS if they do not withdraw from the labour market entirely. Only a minority are thought to switch to the retail sector, such as supermarkets (Skills for Care 2007b), although prior to this information, anecdotal reports have suggested that this is a frequent occurrence. This situation may not be stable since many of the 'people skills' gained in social care are likely to be attractive to a range of employers.

Faced with staff shortages, some employers in the UK have looked to international recruitment as a way of dealing with their staffing problems rather than older workers or to those who may have retired early. While this is not a new phenomenon (Wanless 2006), the advent of the A8 EU accession states (Czech Republic, Estonia, Hungary, Latvia, Lithuania, Poland, Slovakia and Slovenia) has meant that there are new 'sending countries' in addition to traditional sources, such as the Philippines. The long-term impact of this is unknown for such workers whose experiences will test the portability of pension entitlements.

In addition to the initiatives developed by employers, the UK government has also intervened to improve recruitment and retention, with all four UK Care Councils including information on careers in social care on their website and a series of national media advertising campaigns in England aimed at improving the status of social care and attracting more people to work in the area. While much of this work is targeted at young people, with schemes such as Modern Apprentices and Cadets, the government has also sought to improve retention by providing additional funds for training, including increasing the number of places on social work programmes and providing funds to employers to enable their staff to undertake National Vocational Qualifications (NVQs) and to receive induction training. There is some evidence that older people are no longer overtly discriminated against in such initiatives (Mullins 2007; see Box 6.3) but studies of older workers' views about training in social care reveal that they often do not feel that such training is for them.

Box 6.3 Training older workers

Tony Mullins was employed in social care as an assistant social worker and community care worker for 21 years before he embarked on training. He undertook work-based training for three years and then received funding from his employer, a local authority, at the age of 52 to follow the professional qualification in social work. He is now a social worker in the Older People's team.

(*Professional Social Work* 2007: 11)

The lead central government department for health and social care, the English Department of Health, has reported its own recruitment practice in terms of age (Lewis 2007; see Tables 6.4 and 6.5) and it is clear that it too has a long way to go in terms of positive encouragement of older staff, and might be wise to avoid negative comments about other employers.

Table 6.4 Proportion of older workers employed by the Department of Health

	Percentage of staff over 60
31 March 2005	1.0
31 March 2006	1.4
31 March 2007	1.7

Source: Lewis (2007).

Table 6.5 Recruitments to Department of Health aged over 55

	Staff aged 55 and over		Staff aged 60 and over	
	N	%	N	%
2004–2005	5	4	0	0
2005–2006	14	5	3	1
2006–2007	1	1	1	1

Source: Lewis (2007).

Training

In 1998, the White Paper *Modernising Social Services* (Secretary of State for Health 1998, para 5.1) highlighted that 80 per cent of social care staff had no recognized qualifications or training. Gospel and Thompson (2003) found that some older staff working in social care felt that they were too old for training – being the 'wrong side of 50'; and also reported that family commitments presented a barrier to its completion. Among the older workers interviewed in this study, resistance on the part of staff or fear was identified – some did not have the basic skills; others thought they were too old; others feared it might be like 'going back to school' and were worried about being 'tested'. Staff appreciated training that was not based on written work and if they could use a room where they were working (e.g. in a care home) for their studies. Managers too thought it was important that training could be done in the workplace.

Social care employers

No discussion of older workers in social care would be complete without a further reference to the importance of the changing nature of the sector. Recent years have seen changes to the type of businesses in social care, with higher rates of closures among the small independently owned care homes in the UK (Netten et al. 2002), some of which is attributable to the retirement of owners of family businesses and some of which can be attributed to new forms of support, including better home-based services, assistive technology and extra care housing, in line with most older people's preferences to remain at home (Department of Health 2005). However, there has also been a rise in the number of large corporate providers, including multinationals, leading to the invention of the word 'caretelization' (Scourfield 2007). This pattern, whereby the contracting out of care services is followed by consolidation of labour market with concentration under a few providers (Schmid 2003), can also be discerned in other countries in the developed world (Lethbridge 2005). At one level this may bring advantages for older workers since human resources arrangements are likely to be more professionalized and aware of legal frameworks around equal opportunities and employment regulations.

Part of the social care sector may be in good shape compared to others as it is comparatively well prepared for the advent of age regulations in UK (McNair and Flynn 2006: 5). Additionally, within local government and the voluntary sector, equal opportunities policies are common (Department of Work and Pensions 2001). Box 6.4 gives examples where employers have made efforts to recruit older workers and ensure that they are treated fairly.

Box 6.4 Good practice in employment

Age Concern Hull

Age Concern Hull is an independent charity linked to Age Concern England that employs 51 staff and works with several hundred volunteers. Its equal opportunities policy states that: 'As an employer, we genuinely value the wide diversity within our employees; they are judged, not by their age, but according to their ability and skills ...'. Newly appointed staff members complete an anonymized questionnaire on their selection process. Summary data is analysed by management to ensure that the organization's non-discriminatory policies are being implemented effectively.

> 'Age Concern Hull is an equal opportunities organisation. Its policy is to ensure that no one connected with the organisation receives less favourable treatment on the grounds of age, disability, ethnic origin, gender, marital status, race, religious belief, sexual orientation or political allegiance. Harassment of any kind (but specifically on the grounds of age, gender, disability, race or sexual orientation) will be considered a disciplinary offence.'
>
> (Department of Work and Pensions 2001)

Shaw Homes

Shaw Homes employs about 750 staff in 27 nursing homes and residential care homes throughout southern and central England and Wales. It is a not-for-profit organization with charitable status. Around

30 per cent of staff members are aged over 50. St Johns Residential Care Home in the West Midlands of England employs 35 staff, one-third of which are aged over 50 years.

> 'We have a 'person-centred' approach to meeting staff needs. If the need for an ergonomic adjustment arises in relation to a staff members age – we will discuss this and endeavour to make changes in order to retain the skills and expertise of our employee.'
>
> (Department of Work and Pensions 2001)

> 'Shaw Homes finds that advertising flexible working opportunities attracts older workers so it promotes their offer of flexible hours and working conditions to all staff. It reports that older members of staff are sensitive in their support for home residents, that they are reliable and flexible, that they are committed to their work, stay in it for long periods and bring a willingness to work in teams and valuable life skills.'
>
> (Age Positive 2007)

Drawing on a survey conducted for the Department of Work and Pensions and Department of Trade and Industry in 2005, with 214 employers in health and social care in the UK, McNair and Flynn (2006) found that generally the sector has very positive attitudes to older workers (see Box 6.2). While not perfect, it enables them to be flexible in choosing retirement dates, makes it possible for them to stay on after retirement age more than other sectors, and it is more likely than other employers to offer flexible working arrangements. Some employers encourage older workers to stay on after retirement age although there is not much active recruitment of older workers. However, McNair and Flynn (2006: 12) observed that social care employers are more likely to request age details on employment forms than health and other employers and that social care employers are less willing to recruit people above state pension age.

The other main development in social care work is the increase in the number of people employing their own care workers directly. Almost 24,000 people receive direct payments in England (HM Government/Department of Health 2006) and there are almost a further 2,000 recipients in Scotland (Scottish Executive 2006a). Little is known about the characteristics of the workforce supporting them, but it is possible that the intended expansion of direct payments (HM Government/Department of Health 2006) will lead to a growth in the numbers of people operating as 'own account' or self-employed workers in social care. For older workers this may have the advantages of work being flexible and may possibly increase work satisfaction owning to greater autonomy and the ability to provide a more personalized service; however, self-employment has its risks and there may be little or no protection in respect of sickness, injury at work or pension plans. Social care may be emotional labour but it can also involve heavy work such as lifting and handling.

Future trends

There is a move in the UK from seeing the ageing of the social care workforce as simply a matter of concern. Older people are being increasingly viewed not simply as the problem but as part of the solution. As this chapter has shown, social care is a fast-changing sector in the UK, but several factors could affect its activities in the future and thus the workforce profile. The sector has traditionally relied upon a workforce dominated by women who are middle aged and often approaching retirement who possess few professional and educational qualifications; their supply is likely to decline both for demographic reasons and because of women's changing expectations about their options for employment (Cameron et al. 2002). However, at the same time, efforts are being made to widen the base of people attracted to work in social care; for example, mature or older people, men and some minority ethnic groups, so that the workforce is better able to reflect the diversity of the communities it serves (Department of Health/Department for Education and Skills 2006). This may result in social care workers being second career or second or even third chance workers, perhaps with a variety of employments and casual work who may be better able to argue that flexibility in paid work needs to be appreciated and rewarded. Otherwise, while greater casualization may provide the opportunity for low paid or lowly pensioned people to earn extra income, it will sustain low pay and poverty in later life.

Much will also be affected by future needs for care within the older population and other groups who need support, although there is not always a direct relationship between the need for care and the profile of the labour force (Hussein and Manthorpe 2005). Throughout Europe, the increase in the number of countries in which 'cash for care' options are available may have further impacts on the labour force (Ungerson and Yeandle 2006). Originally, people receiving direct payments in the UK were not allowed to use them to pay members of the family and friends but this has been changed. This may lead to a blurring of the boundaries between paid care and so-called informal care and older people may find low-paid social care work in the grey or unofficial economy a short-term solution to financial pressures.

In England, both the Children's Workforce Development Council (CWDC) and Skills for Care (SfC) have been working towards the development of new types of worker; that is, workers whose roles are a hybrid between health and social care, or who are 'experts by experience' (i.e. they have personal experience of using a particular service), workers who help people 'navigate' between different services or advocate on their behalf. For many social care workers in later life, these roles may be appealing and may make the most of their skills and experiences. Whether these changes will lead to the development of new and fulfilling roles for workers in later life, as well as offering an improved service and increased choice for people using these services, is something that will only emerge with time.

References

Age Positive (undated) *Case Study: Wokingham District Council* (www.agepositive.gov.uk).

Anderson, T., Forth, J., Metcalf, H. and Kirby, S. (2001) *The Gender Pay Gap: Final Report to the Women and Equality Unit.* London: The Cabinet Office.

Anxo, D. and Fagan, C. (2001) Service employment: a gender perspective, in D. Anxo and D. Storrie (eds) *The Job Creation Potential of the Service Sector in Europe*, pp. 89–111. Luxembourg: Office for Official Publications of the European Communities.

Balloch, S., McLean, J. and Fisher, M. (1999) *Social Services: Working Under Pressure*. Bristol: The Policy Press.

Barnes, H. and Taylor, R. (2006) *Work, Saving and Retirement Among Ethnic Minorities: A Qualitative Study*, Research Report No. 396. London: Department for Work and Pensions.

Beishon, S., Virdee, S. and Hagell, A. (1995) *Nursing in a Multi-ethnic NHS.* London: Policy Studies Institute.

Bennett, J., Davey, B. and Harris, R. (2007) *Nurses Working in Mid-life.* London: Nursing Research Unit (www.kcl.ac.uk/content/1/c6/01/69/82/MidLifeFinalReport.pdf).

Butt, J., Gorbach, P. and Ahmed, B. (1991) *Equally Fair: A Report on Social Services Departments' Development, Implementation and Monitoring of Services for the Black and Minority Ethnic Community.* London: National Institute for Social Work Research Unit/Race Equality Unit/Social Services Research Group.

Cameron, C. and Moss, P. (2007) *Care Work in Europe: Current Undertakings and Future Directions*. Abingdon: Routledge.

Cameron, C., Mooney, A. and Moss, P. (2002) The child care workforce: current conditions and future directions, *Critical Social Policy*, 22(4): 572–95.

Cameron, C., Moss, P. and Owen, C. (1999) *Men in the Nursery: Gender and Caring Work*. London: Paul Chapman Publishing.

Care Council for Wales (undated) *The Social Care Workforce in Wales: Themes and Trends*. Cardiff: Care Council for Wales (www.ccwales.org.uk/DesktopDefault.aspx?tabid=130).

Christie, A. (1998) Is social work a 'non-traditional' occupation for men? *British Journal of Social Work*, 28(4): 491–510.

Christie, A. (2006) Negotiating the uncomfortable intersections between gender and professional identities in social work, *Critical Social Policy*, 26(2): 390–411.

Clark, K. and Drinkwater, S. (2007) *Ethnic Minorities in the Labour Market: Dynamics and Diversity*. Bristol: The Policy Press (www.jrf.org.uk/bookshop/eBooks/1986-ethnic-minorities-employment.pdf).

Commission for Social Care Inspection (2006) *The State of Social Care in England 2005–2006*. London: Commission for Social Care Inspection (www.csci.org.uk/pdf/state_of_social_care_05–06_1.pdf).

Commission for Social Care Inspection (2007) *What is Social Care?* (www.csci.org.uk/about_us/what_is_social_care.aspx: accessed 29 July 2008).

Conley, H.M. (2003) Temporary work in the public services: implications for equal opportunities, *Gender Work & Organization*, 10(4): 455–77.

Cross, S. and Bagilhole, B. (2002) Girls' jobs for the boys? Men, masculinity and non-traditional occupations, *Gender, Work & Organization*, 9(2): 204–26.

Davey, B. (2002) Management progression and ambition: women and men in social work, *Research Policy and Planning*, 20(2): 21–34.

Davey, B., Kearney, P. and Rosen, G. (2000) Equalling the opportunity of a management career, in E. Harlow and J. Lawlor (eds) *Management, Social Work and Change*, pp. 93–115. Aldershot: Ashgate.

Davidson, K., Daly, T. and Arber, S. (2003) Older men, social integration and organisational activities, *Social Policy and Society*, 2(2): 81–89.

Department of Health (2005) *Independence, Well-being and Choice: Our Vision for the Future of Social Care for Adults in England, Cm 6499*. Norwich: The Stationery Office (TSO). (www.dh.gov.uk/assetRoot/04/10/64/78/04106478.pdf).

Department of Health Social Services and Public Safety (2006) *Personal Social Services: Development and Training Strategy 2006–2016*. Belfast: Department of Health Social Services and Public Safety (www.dhsspsni.gov.uk/pss-development-training-trategy-2006–2016.pdf).

Department of Health/Department for Education and Skills (2006) *Options for Excellence: Building the Social Care Workforce of the Future*. London: Department of Health (www.everychildmatters.gov.uk/_files/C0A219467E447BCF511284 CDAB479F93.pdf)).

Department of Work and Pensions (2001) *Good Practice in the Recruitment and Retention of Older Workers: Case Studies*. Nottingham: DWP Publications (www.workandpensions.gov.uk/asd/asd5/rports2005–2006/agepos16(2).pdf).

Eborall, C. (2003) *The State of the Social Care Workforce in England: Volume 1 of the first Annual Report of the TOPSS England Workforce Intelligence Unit, 2003*. Leeds: TOPSS England (www.nmds-sc.org.uk/repository.asp?section=12).

Eborall, C. (2005) *The State of the Social Care Workforce 2004: The second Skills Research & Intelligence annual report*. Leeds: Skills for Care (www.nmds-sc.org.uk/repository.asp?section=11).

Esping-Andersen, G. (1999) *Social Foundations of Post Industrial Economies*. Oxford: Oxford University Press.

Ewijk, H.v., Hens, H., Lammersen, G. and Moss, P. (2002) *WP3. Mapping of Care Services and the Care Workforce. Consolidated Report*. Utrecht: Netherlands Institute of Care and Welfare.

Eyers, I. and Bryan, K. (2006) Professionalising the care of older people: transforming the workforce, *Quality in Ageing*, 7(4): 37–45.

Forder, J., Knapp, M., Hardy, B. et al. (2004) Prices, contracts and motivations: institutional arrangements in domiciliary care, *Policy & Politics*, 32: 207–22.

Francis, J. and Netten, A. (2003) *Home Care Workers: Careers, Commitments and Motivations*, Discussion paper No. 2053. Canterbury: Personal Social Services Research Unit (www.pssru.ac.uk/pdf/dp2053.pdf).

Gospel, H. and Thompson, M. (2003) *The Role and Impact of the Statutory Framework for Training in the Social Care Sector*, Research Report No. 495. Nottingham: DfES Publications (www.dfes.gov.uk/research/data/uploadfiles/ RR495.pdf).

Government Equalities Office (2008) *Gender Pay Gap* (www.equalities.gov.uk/ women_work/pay.htm: accessed 29 July 2008).

Grimshaw, D. (2002) *Qualitative Research on Firms' Adjustments to the Minimum Wage*. Manchester: European Work and Employment Research Centre (www.lowpay.gov.uk/lowpay/research/pdf/grim.pdf).

Grimshaw, D. and Carroll, M. (2006) Adjusting to the national minimum wage: constraints and incentives to change in six low-paying sectors, *Industrial Relations Journal*, 37(1): 22–47.

Grimshaw, D. and Rubery, J. (2007) *Undervaluing Women's Work*, Working Paper No. 53. Manchester: Equal Opportunities Commission (www.eoc.org.uk/PDF/WP53_undervaluing_womens_work.pdf).

Hancock, R., Wittenberg, R., Pickard, L. et al. (2007) *Paying for Long-term Care for Older People in the UK: Modelling the Costs and Distributional Effects of a Range of Options*, PSSRU Discussion Paper No. 2336/2. London: London School of Economics (www.pssru.ac.uk/pdf/dp2336_2.pdf).

Hillmann, F. (2005) Migrants' care work in private households, or: the strength of bilocal and transnational ties as a last(ing) resource in global migration, in B. Pfau-Effinger and B. Geissler (eds) *Care and Social Integration in European Societies*, pp. 93–112. Bristol: The Policy Press.

HM Government/Department of Health (2006) *Our Health, Our Care, Our Say: A New Direction for Community Services*, Cm 6737. London: Department of Health (www.dh.gov.uk/assetRoot/04/12/74/59/04127459.pdf).

Hussein, S. and Manthorpe, J. (2005) An international review of the long-term care workforce policies and shortages, *Journal of Aging & Social Policy*, 17(4): 75–94.

Hwalek, M. and Essenmacher, V. (2005) *Older Workers in Direct Care: A Labor Force Expansion Study*. Detroit, MI: SPEC Associates (www.bjbc.org/content/docs/OperationABLEFinalReport112905.pdf).

Knapp, M., Hardy, B. and Forder, J. (2001) Commissioning for quality: ten years of social care markets in England, *Journal of Social Policy*, 30(2): 283–306.

Kosniewski, K. and Hwalek, M. (2006) *Older Workers in Direct Care: A Labor Force Expansion Study. Executive Summary*. Washington, DC: Better Jobs Better Care (www.bjbc.org/content/docs/ExecSummary_op_Able_FINALCOLOR8–06.pdf).

Learning and Skills Council (2006) *National Employers Skills Survey 2005: Main Report*. Coventry: Learning and Skills Council (www.research.lsc.gov.uk/LSC+Research/published/ness/).

Lethbridge, J. (2005) *Care Services in Europe*. London: Public Services International Research Unit (PSIRU) (www.psiru.org/reports/_Toc96224874).

Lewis, I. (2007) *Departments: Older Workers. Hansard: Written Answer to Questions*, 4 July 2007, Col. 1102W. London: House of Commons.

Local Authority Workforce Intelligence Group (2006) *Adult, Children and Young People Local Authority Social Care Workforce Survey 2005*. London: Local Government Association (www.lga.gov.uk/Briefing.asp?lSection=0&id=SX1282-A783CEF3).

Low Pay Commission (2007) *National Minimum Wage: Low Pay Commission Report 2007*. London: Low Pay Commission (www.lowpay.gov.uk/lowpay/report/pdf/6828-DTi-Low_Pay_Complete.pdf).

Lupton, B. (2006) Explaining men's entry into female-concentrated occupations: issues of masculinity and social class, *Gender, Work & Organization*, 13(2): 103–28.

Machin, S. and Manning, A. (2002) *The Structure of Wages in What Should be a Competitive Labour Market*, Discussion Paper No. CEPDP0532. London: Centre for Economic Performance (www.cep.lse.ac.uk/pubs/download/DP0532.pdf).

Machin, S., Manning, A. and Rahman, L. (2002) *Where the Minimum Wage Bites Hard: The Introduction of the UK National Minimum Wage to a Low Wage Sector*, Discussion Paper No. CEPDP0544. London: Centre for Economic Performance (www.cep.lse.ac.uk/pubs/download/DP0544.pdf).

McLean, J. (2003) Men as minority: men employed in statutory social care work, *Journal of Social Work*, 3(1): 45–68.

McNair, S. and Flynn, M. (2006) *Managing an Ageing Workforce in Health and Social Care*. London: Department for Work and Pensions (www.agepositive.gov.uk/publications/Man_Age_HealthSoc_v5.pdf).

Mullins, T. (2007) Interview: life begins at 55½, *Professional Social Work* (September): 11.

Netten, A., Darton, R. and Williams, J. (2002) *The Rate, Causes and Consequences of Home Closures*. Canterbury: Personal Social Services Research Unit (www.pssru.ac.uk/pdf/dp1741~2.pdf).

Office for National Statistics (2002) *Social Focus in Brief: Ethnicity*. London: Office for National Statistics (www.statistics.gov.uk/downloads/theme_social/social_focus_in_brief/ethnicity/ethnicity.pdf).

Office for National Statistics (2006) *Social Trends 37*. London: Office for National Statistics (www.statistics.gov.uk/downloads/theme_social/Social_Trends37/Social_Trends_37.pdf).

Office for National Statistics (2007) *Population Estimates: UK Population Grows to 60.6 million*. London: Office for National Statistics.

Office for National Statistics (undated) *2006 Annual Survey of Hours and Earnings (ASHE) Analysis by Occupation*. London: Office for National Statistics.

Owen, D. (2001) *Profile of Black and Minority Ethnic Groups in the UK*. Warwick: Centre for Research in Ethnic Relations (www2.warwick.ac.uk/fac/cross_fac/healthatwarwick/publications/occasional/ethnicprofile.pdf).

Palese, A., Oliverio, F., Girardo, M.F., Fabbro, E. and Saiani, L. (2004) Difficulties and workload of foreign caregivers: a descriptive analysis, *Diversity in Health and Social Care*, 1(1): 31–38.

Platt, D. (2007) *The Status of Social Care: A Review 2007*. London: Department of Health (www.dh.gov.uk/en/Publicationsandstatistics/Publications/PublicationsPolicyAndGuidance/DH_074217).

Robinson, J. and Banks, P. (2005) *The Business of Caring: King's Fund Inquiry into Care Services in London*. London: King's Fund (www.kingsfund.org.uk/resources/publications/the_business_of.html).

Rolfe, H., Metcalf, H., Anderson, T. and Meadows, P. (2003) *Recruitment and Retention of Childcare, Early years and Playworkers: Research Study*. DfES Research Report No. 409. London: National Institute of Economic and Social Research (www.dfes.gov.uk/research/data/uploadfiles/RR409.doc).

Schmid, H. (2003) Rethinking the policy of contracting out Social Services to non-governmental organizations, *Public Management Review*, 5(3): 307–23.

Scottish Executive (2006a) *Direct Payments Scotland, 2006*. Edinburgh: Scottish Executive (www.scotland.gov.uk/Resource/Doc/149651/0039854.pdf).

Scottish Executive (2006b) *Scotland's Social Services Labour Market: 2nd report of National Workforce Group*. Edinburgh: Scottish Executive (www.socialworkscotland.org.uk/resources/cp-wf/2ndLabourMarketReport.pdf).

Scourfield, P. (2007) Are there reasons to be worried about the 'caretelization' of residential care? *Critical Social Policy*, 27(2): 155–80.

Secretary of State for Health (1998) *Modernising Social Services: Promoting Independence, Improving Protection, Raising Standards*, Cm 4169. London: The Stationery Office (TSO) (www.archive.official-documents.co.uk/document/cm41/4169/4169.htm).

Skills for Care (2007a) *NMDS-SC Briefing. Issue 1 Overview – an Oasis in the Data Desert*. Leeds: Skills for Care (www.nmds-sc.org.uk/news.asp).

Skills for Care (2007b) *NMDS-SC Briefing. Issue 2 Turnover and Vacancy Rates*. Leeds: Skills for Care (www.nmds-sc.org.uk/news.asp).

Ungerson, C. (2000) Thinking about the production and consumption of long term care in Britain: does gender still matter? *Journal of Social Policy*, 29(4): 623–43.

Ungerson, C. and Yeandle, S. (2006) *Cash for Care in Developed Welfare States*. Basingstoke: Palgrave Macmillan.

Walker, A. (1997) *Combating Age Barriers in Employment: European Research Report*. Luxembourg: Office of Official Publications of the European Communities.

Wanless, D. (2006) *Securing Good Care for Older People: Taking a Long-term View*. London: King's Fund (www.kingsfund.org.uk/resources/publications/securing_good.html).

Women & Equality Unit (2006) What is the pay gap and why does it exist? London.

7 An overview of developing a mature workforce

Patrick Grattan

This chapter is informed by the experiences of The Age and Employment Network (TAEN). Formerly known as the Third Age Employment Network, it was started in 1998 in the United Kingdom (UK) as a not-for-profit enterprise and registered charity to find ways of making the labour market operate better for people in mid- and later life. Its origins lay in the frustrations of many people aged over 50 who felt that they had been put on the scrap heap well before their time.

With the growing interest in the subject of age and employment, TAEN flourished and has become a leading centre of expertise with an influential role in public policy. Its members now include over 250 organizations, made up of employers, training providers, colleges, recruitment and employment agencies, voluntary and community organizations, public agencies at national, regional and local level, individuals, unions, employment lawyers, think tanks and others.

This chapter looks at the contribution which government and public agencies, employers, unions and individuals have made in the last few years in response to demographic change and its major impact on patterns of life and work. It also examines the innovative approaches that will be needed if we are to stay ahead and profit from the opportunity of longer lives.

Go back to 2000 and we were still living in an era that Adair Turner and his colleagues on the Pensions Commission were subsequently to describe as a 'fool's paradise' (DWP 2004). It is true that the new Labour Government in 1997 had started to take an interest in age and employment. New Deal 50 plus was a ground-breaking welfare to work programme which was introduced in 1999. In the same year a Code of Good Practice on age and employment was issued (DEE 1988). However, all this hardly registered on the Richter scale of political and business interest. Youth was a *leitmotif* of New Labour and ending youth unemployment an understandable central objective.

With benefit of hindsight, it is curious that the 25-year fall in employment levels of people aged over 50 starting in the 1970s did not attract more attention at the time. The dramatic rise in numbers of people, especially men, categorized as sick or disabled from the early 1990s likewise passed unnoticed. Political and business commentators remained glued to the unemployment rate (the numbers registered as unemployed), even though it was becoming less and less meaningful as a barometer of the labour market.

However, by the mid-1990s the 30-year decline in employment of over-50s men had halted. Since the late 1990s there has been a steady growth in employment for all ages and in particular of the over-50s. Two-thirds of the growth of the UK labour force to its current all-time high has been made up of people aged over 50, including the fastest recorded growth among those over state pension age (Table 7.1).

Table 7.1 Workforce and employment rate 1997–2006 by age and gender

Employment All	18–24	25–49	50–SPA	Post-SPA
1997	3.3m	16.6m	5.2m	0.8m
2006	3.5m	17.2m	6.5m	1.2m
Change 1997–2006	+0.2m	**+0.6m**	**+1.3m**	+0.4m
Employment Rate All				
1997	66%	79%	64%	8%
2006	65%	**82%**	**71%**	11%
Change 1997–2006	–1%	+3%	+7%	+3%
Employment Male				
1997	1.7m	9.0m	3.1m	0.3m
2006	1.8m	9.2m	3.8m	0.4m
Change 1997–2006	+0.1m	+0.2m	+0.7m	0.1m
Employment Female				
1997	1.5m	7.6m	2.0m	0.5m
2006	1.6m	8.0m	2.6m	0.8m
Change 1997–2006	+0.1m	+0.4m	+0.6m	+0.3m

Source: Labour Force Survey Summer (2006).

The population in the 50–64 age cohort has been rising in this period. This means that of the 1.4 million increase in workers aged over 50, some 900,000, represents absorption of the increased numbers of older people in the labour force, while the additional 400,000 represent an increase in the employment rate of people over the age of 50 from 64 per cent to almost 71 per cent.

There has also been a change in the gender balance of the workforce. Employment of women of all ages increased. The rate of increase of the over-50s women was slower – if the growth had been as rapid as the growth among the under-50s, there would be 250,000 more women over 50 in work by now. An interesting future exploration will be to see how patterns of work among the next age cohort of women are influenced by their career experience as younger women, which often have been quite different from that of their mothers' generation.

So what has driven this turn around?

Employer action

Action by employers has clearly contributed to the improvement in the employment rate of the over-50s. By definition more people are being retained or recruited in their 50s and 60s than was the case in the 1990s. The cost of early voluntary redundancy (one of the main drivers for earlier retirement ages in the 1980s and 1990s) has become prohibitive for over-stretched pension funds, although exception is still made for a minority of senior executives as an aid to succession management.

A considerable body of good practice in all-age recruitment and retention has built up. The government's Age Positive campaign, run by the Department of Work and Pensions, has a wide range of case studies of what employers have done to identify the age profile of their workforce, age neutral recruitment policies and other procedures and raise the modest percentage of their workforce drawn from the over-50s population. Leading employers increased the proportion of their workforce aged over 50 from under 10 per cent to around 20 per cent in relatively short periods by encouraging retention and removing incentives to early retirement. This included both large and small businesses – see www.agepositive.gov.uk. Many larger businesses already committed to active policies on gender, race and disability worked with the Employers Forum on Age (EFA 2008) (see www.efa.org.uk). This has included both public and private sector businesses.

In some sectors, such as retail and financial services, there is a much greater realization of the connection between the age profile of customer-facing employees and the customers. The fact that 80 per cent of the wealth of the UK is owned by people over 50 should be enough to concentrate the mind of many businesses. Large retailers in particular have realized that their 7 x 24 and seasonal work patterns fit well with the desire of many older people for flexible, seasonal and part-time work.

The change should not, however, be exaggerated. The gap between statements of intent and day-to-day practice remains great. In large businesses the good intentions of corporate human resource departments do not translate overnight into operational practice by line management. Awareness of demographic change is limited. Senior management remains convinced that older workers cost more, are less productive and are sick more often. No amount of direct factual evidence to the contrary makes much dent in entrenched stereotypical thinking.

The views of the Confederation of British Industry (CBI) (2004) on retirement ages and legislation carry an implicit assumption that older workers are more problematic to manage than younger workers. Yet the evidence on the commercial benefit to companies that have broadened the age profile of their workforce is forceful. No company has yet reported disastrous consequences of employing more people aged over 50; rather, they have reported a win-win situation for employees and employer.

The position of the majority of UK businesses that have less than 50 employees is paradoxical. They are less 'ageist' than large businesses and public sector employers where grade=status=age rules. They will employ the best person for the job without a thought for age. At the same time, they may be unconscious of age legislation and such matters as fixed retirement ages.

The impact of demographics

This has been an important influence on employment. Only in the past few years have we become aware of the speed in the growth of life expectancy. The Pensions Commission administered a reality check in its first report in October 2004. The improvement in mortality rates has been accelerating. But forecasts of future life expectancy have been accelerating even faster. It seems as if actuaries and pension managers are permanently running to catch up.

Policy issues on age and employment are ill-served by the evidence base and confusion surrounding life expectancy forecasts (TAEN 2007b). Average life expectancy at birth and average life expectancy at age 65 are frequently confused (average life expectancy at birth factors in the 1 in 10 of people who die by the age of 65). The government is frustrated because people do not believe the statistics on life expectancy, and therefore do not act to prepare for longer lives.

Individual attitudes to mortality risk depend on individual risk not collective risk. The consequences of dying sooner for the individual are not symmetrical with the consequences of living to 100. So it is understandable that even those who are aware that life expectancy for 65-year-olds is rising well into the 80s work on the assumption that it will not apply to them.

Health is improving. It is regularly observed that today's 70-year-olds are yesterday's 60-year-olds and are behaving accordingly. Deaths from cancer and heart condition amongst those in their 60s and 70s have both fallen dramatically in the last 10 years. The scope for more years of working life, whether paid or unpaid, is enhanced compared with previous generations. The duration of healthy old age is increasing roughly in parallel with actual life expectancy.

In 10 years of New Labour, inequality between different socio-economic groups has not reduced. Most indicators of educational attainment, income and asset accumulation, health or life expectancy have not narrowed. Some have widened. The poor, including lone parents and older people, have become less poor and have been aided in this by the tax credit system, but the better off have continued to become better off at a faster rate (Dorling et al. 2007). As long as there is a difference of up to 8 years in average life expectancy between two neighbourhoods, this will have a profound impact on the politics of retirement, pensions and work.

Those who retire earliest (because of good final salary pension schemes) are the best off in retirement, while those who retire latest (manual and unqualified workers with no savings who carry on until state pension age) are least well off in retirement. It seems perverse that those who retire earliest are rewarded for that. It would make better economic and social sense if those who worked longer were rewarded more for their efforts in retirement.

Declining retirement incomes

The sight of expected payouts from pension and other savings for retirement plummeting in the last five years has certainly influenced the employment rate of the over-50s and indeed the over-65s. It is likely that it outstrips the impact of all other factors, be they government policy, age discrimination legislation or employer actions.

The pension world has changed since 2000. There has been a recovery of financial markets but this is more than outweighed by the negative impact of building in longer life expectancy to pension payment calculations. It is widely expected that the era of final salary pension schemes is ending and will not be rebuilt, unless it is for a small elite of directors and public sector workers. The most common alternative is defined contribution schemes. On current calculations they yield a retirement income half what they would have done five years ago because of lower returns and increased life expectancy. It changes one's perspective to working longer to know that the pension scheme you thought would give you £12,000 a year will now only give you £6,000 (TAEN 2008).

In addition, the move from defined benefit to defined contribution pensions in the private sector has replaced a system that rewarded early retirement with a system that puts most of the risk on the individual employee. It thus creates incentives to continue working and building a pension fund for retirement income that may have to stretch over a longer period.

There is a new perspective on pension risks. Most people with occupational pensions genuinely thought that they were risk-free. It is only in the past few years that we have discovered that there is no such thing as a risk-free pension scheme, despite the creation of the Pension Protection Fund. Confidence in traditional pension saving businesses is at an all-time low and confidence in government to deliver a secure national pension saving scheme is not high.

The high rates of return up to 2000 shielded us from the reality of pension economics – they allowed the pensions industry to take a handsome cut for running our pensions while still giving most of us on such schemes a good deal. Lower returns have brought home that around half the total value of a private pension scheme is used up on remunerating the financial adviser and pension manager, leaving insufficient to pay an acceptable level of pension. The economics of small- or average-sized pension schemes run by the private sector, as opposed to the government, no longer make sense. Hence the flight, for those with the resources, into investing in property.

Declining State pensions

In the early days of the Labour administration, there was widespread support for the move to a means-tested state pension system. Concentrating public funds on those who most needed support made sense. The system of a standard state pension, more or less adequate to support a simple life in retirement, had operated since Beveridge and the 1940s (Beveridge 1942), and was reckoned to have run its course.

The new selective benefits and pension route has proved a classic example of a good policy purpose beset by delivery problems such as:

- administrative machinery that could not cope;
- incomprehensibility to the general public and specifically to those who most need it;
- spread of means-testing on a massive scale that had not been envisaged;
- the decline of the basic pension to a risible level relative to average earnings.

The options are to stand by the New Labour means-tested model or to revert to the universal model of state safety net for those who do not have their own resources. One way or the other there is a transitional period from dependence on the state to self-reliance. Savers are either penalized for saving when the universal pension is taxed away, or the means-tested pension recipient is penalized when a means-tested benefit is phased out for those with savings.

From welfare into work

The government's welfare to work policies have been a success story and a contributor, along with macro-economic stability, to the highest employment rate the UK has known, well ahead of most OECD countries. However, our assessment is that government employment policies have been only a modest contributor for older people, as compared to the overall impact of economic stability and growth.

When New Deal 50 plus was introduced in 1999, the government decided not to make it compulsory (DWP 2008). As a voluntary programme with an 'employment credit' paid directly to individuals who returned to work in a modestly paid job, it was a great success in 2000–03 with 100,000 people aged over 50 taking up the option. Since 2003 it has languished and now it is nearly extinct.

The programme to help people leave incapacity benefit (IB) is important for older people. Half the 2.7 million people on IB are aged over 50 years. In the early tests, there was encouraging evidence that the intensive help was equally successful with all ages of IB claimants (it was in the main trialled with people moving on to this benefit) and that longer-term claimants who volunteered were also successful. More recently, it seems that the combined factors of age and disability are proving tough barriers for the over-50s. The government has put off implementing the programme for most of the existing 1.4 million people over 50 who have been claiming the benefit for some time. It is therefore not likely that this is going to be a major contributor to improving the employment rate (ELMR 2007).

The impact of age legislation

Up to the year 2000 there was little or no prospect of age legislation comparable to existing legislation on gender, 'race' and disability discrimination, despite evidence that age is the commonly experienced barrier to opportunity in work and learning (Ray et al. 2005). However, in late 2000 the UK Government agreed to an EU Equal Treatment Directive on race, disability, age, religion/belief and sexual orientation. It took the lead in arguing that age legislation had major complexity and that member states should have six years in which to transpose the Directive to national law, unlike the other topics that had to be actioned within a three-year period.

These 6 years were up at the end of 2006 and UK age legislation is now in force (*The Employment Equality (Age) Regulations 2006* Statutory Instrument 2006 No. 1031). Its introduction generated a high level of public interest. It has certainly helped raise awareness to a different level from what it would have been without legislation. Many employers, mainly the larger ones, have taken action to adjust their human resource management procedures to reduce the risks of a legal challenge to age-based practices. Huge numbers of others, of course, have not done so and have not heard of the legislation.

The effectiveness of age legislation will be much like other equalities acts. They are not a magic potion. Employment indicators on race or gender have moved only modestly years after legislation was passed. But that does not mean that the legislation has been pointless. The world is a different place as a result of such legislation and it is already different as a result of the 2006 UK age law.

It is often asked whether age discrimination is different from other forms of discrimination. This will be relevant with the new Commission on Equality and Human Rights (CEHR 2008) started in late 2007, replacing the existing Equal Opportunities Commission, Commission for Racial Equality and Disability Rights Commission, begins to demonstrate its responsibility for the three new equality strands including age. An obvious observation is that age changes with time while other characteristics do not.

What the work on legislation has shown is that, despite widespread experience of age-based barriers and their impact on people's lives, there is less public involvement than in issues of 'race', gender or disability. Response to government consultations has been limited. There is nothing like the broad front of disability organizations that worked so hard in the 1990s to achieve disability legislation and that continue to work on its improvement. Many of those whose prospects are curtailed by age-based decisions accept it as their lot or conclude that they have 'had their turn'. The case for legislation on age has been driven as much by the economic imperative for change as by the demand for equal treatment. In this the balance is different from the existing equalities legislation.

Looking ahead

The next question is whether this momentum, driven by longer lives, pension economics, government policies, employers' skills needs and the demand for choice about when and how the transition from work to retirement takes place, will continue.

The government has stated its ambition to increase the employment rate from the current 75 per cent for working age (16–60/65) people, to 80 per cent (DWP 2005). This requires an increase of one million people aged over 50 including people over pension age in work, and one million people moving from Incapacity Benefit (of whom half may be aged over 50) and back into work (DWP and DIUS 2007).

The target for people aged over 50 should be achievable, unless there is a major recession. It will be less easy to achieve the movement of one million people off Incapacity Benefit and, on current policies, this seems unlikely to happen.

So much further innovation by government, employers and individuals will be needed if we are to see the increase in employment in midlife and later working life sustained. The rest of this chapter examines these challenges.

The corporate status syndrome – the variable career pattern

Status is important to organizations and individuals. It is also a huge barrier to more flexible views on when and how we do various things at various stages of our lives.

An intrinsic and healthy part of working life is the ambition to increase earnings, to compete and advance up a career and power ladder. It is hard to imagine that this could be entirely separated from status, grade and age. Most of us need to earn more; choice over work-life balance and lifestyle is the privilege of a small minority.

Yet, implicit in demographic change and longer working lives is a more fluid situation. Changing pension and tax rules will make it easier to mix and match work and leisure and downshift without ending working life. In the United States of America (USA) about a third of all people take a bridging job between their main career and full retirement.

There is a great deal of talk about flexible working in the UK. The evidence so far shows that there has been limited movement (ONS 2006). Those who engage in job shares, part-time working, career breaks or study leave are seen as less committed and ambitious, even though there are many examples showing that these are win-win arrangements for business and employees.

We have a long way to travel to diminish the importance of hierarchies and create what we have called in Figure 7.1 the 'roller coaster' careers. These ideas are profoundly counter-cultural in large public and private sector businesses. But there are common characteristics among some people (certainly not all) in the second half of their careers which could push along the shift in corporate culture:

Figure 7.1 Life stages: 'good' work, 'bad' work

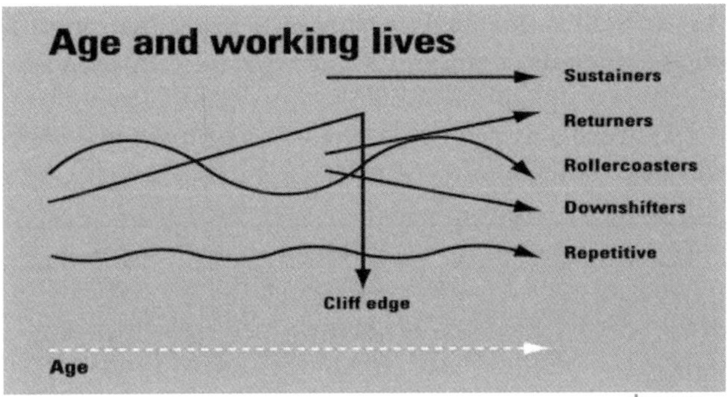

Source: Figure reproduced with permission from TAEN.

- a desire to get back to 'front-line work', doing something practical, making something, as opposed to the years spent in people management and organizational change;
- a greater interest in flexible working and a more balanced view of the role of work alongside the other dimensions of life;
- a more settled view of where we want to get to and what we want to get out of working life – perhaps a realistic acceptance of our potential;
- a strong attachment to the social role of working life;
- a reduction, for some, of the financial pressures of bringing up a family and paying a mortgage.

A precondition for making the labour market work well for all ages is that we press on with changing standard corporate and personal career culture. This means job opportunities in all occupational sectors, good-quality work and rewards. Otherwise a more pessimistic view may come true: older workers slogging on in predominantly low-wage, low-skill jobs with few opportunities to advance.

The government's role

The hazard is that the government will take the achievement of longer working life and later retirement for granted. Increased employment of over-50s has progressed very nicely in the past eight years with limited intervention by government (see Table 7.2) Government programmes that could bolster longer working lives are low down the expenditure pecking order. The reason is evident from Table 7.2 which shows that the shortfall in the employment rate is smaller and narrowing faster than most other target groups such as some ethnic minorities, lone parents and disabled people.

Table 7.2 Difference between target group employment rate and all-age employment rates, UK data

	1997	2006
50-SPA	–7%	–4%
Lone parents	–24%	–16%
Ethnic minorities	–17%	–15%
Disabled people	–27%	–21%
Unskilled	–20%	–28%

Source: ONS (2006) Centre for Economic and Social Inclusion.

Over a quarter of the UK workforce is employed in the public sector. The decision reached in October 2005 with public sector unions to retain the pension age of 60 for all existing employees, while understandable, creates an unsustainable gulf between the public and private sector. It seems inevitable that public and private sector pensions will need to be more closely aligned.

It will also be for government to make a success of the new legislation on age discrimination. This means backing it up with clear guidance and good dispute resolution procedures. The Commission on Equality and Human Rights must be a high-quality and resourced body to promote the legislation, provide advice to the general public and to employers, and support redress for those who have suffered from unacceptable employment practices. There must also be pressure for change in the recruitment industry which remains strongly focused on the 25–45-year-old age group.

Personal barriers and dignity

Sustaining the momentum of a better job market for older people also demands culture change for many individuals. This is tricky territory, touching on the rights and responsibilities of the individual and whether these change with age.

To 20-year-olds we say – go out and do temporary work, gain any kind of experience (it's all good for you), don't do nothing. Get a foot in the door and work on the principle that one thing can lead to another.

What should we expect of over-50s? It is clear that those who are most flexible about what they are prepared to do are the most likely to get back into work. Those who start by defining everything they are not prepared to do or what they are owed because of their age are least likely to find a new role. The reality is that age does not confer special status. Enthusiasm and commitment to turn a hand to whatever needs to be done work best.

At the same time people deserve to have jobs that use their skills and experience. Older people should not have to accept under-employment just because of their age. Many of the most frustrated non-workers in their 50s and 60s are the most qualified. They know that lack of management and professional skills is always cited as one of the key shortages facing British business. Yet, their chances of getting back into a management job comparable to their last job are still close to zero. They know that, despite the progress in the employment rate described above, putting their date of birth on the CV is fatal.

Duration out of work easily becomes a self-fulfilling and self-reinforcing barrier with the passage of time. In theory, a few years' break in employment could be seen as a stimulus to a new career with a new and fresh perspective. Instead, a period away from the workforce means not getting an interview.

These are not easy issues to resolve but progress is needed to free up the labour market so that those who have been formed by their initial training 30 years ago can respond to today's labour market. In summary, the way forward has to be a subtle mix on the part of the jobseeker, aiming for jobs that make good use of skills and experience but not ruling too much out, at least as a stepping-stone.

The role of career advice and training

Possibly the greatest contribution to building a thriving job market and careers in later working life is to unlock the potential of lifelong career advice and training. This is where we lag most in responding to demographic change. Post-school and adult learning activity is dominated by the task of equipping young people for adult life and careers. Once launched on working life few people will have much exposure to formal learning and qualifications again. The model of foundation learning and training up to age 19 or the early 20s to last a 40–50-year working lifetime is no longer fit for purpose.

Individual choice rather than force of circumstance should drive successful adaptation to longer and varied working lives. But this requires a change in the world of career advice. It should be as natural for a 40- or 50-year-old person to seek career advice as for an 18-year-old.

To undertake reskilling as a step to a new career also requires a reasonable assurance of a job at the end of it. There is no point in dedicating effort and resources to training only to find at the end that it is no easier to get a job because of age and/or lack of prior experience.

A test for all of us over the next few years is whether we shall see this change take place. In December 2005 the Leitch Review on Adult Skills (Her Majesty's Treasury 2006) set out an ambitious set of targets for adult qualifications. They were described as essential if the UK is to be internationally competitive. But they will require resources, in competition with the higher education and schools, both of which have pressing needs.

It is not widely realized that the share of adults, qualifications gained by the over-40s needs to rise from less than 5 per cent to around 30 per cent if there is to be any hope of meeting skills targets. This requires a formidable transformation by employers and individuals. It requires a qualifications system that makes sense for workers in mid career and for employers.

Quality of work and work environment

The final field of innovation is quality of work and work environment (TAEN 2007a). This covers:

- good operational management that underpins job satisfaction (the largest single reason for quitting or not returning, especially in the public sector, is dissatisfaction with management and frequent reorganizations and initiatives);
- the potential to advance, as a *quid pro quo*, for accepting an entry-level job at a modest level;
- proactive occupational health policies, job design and work environments to promote good health in mid- and later life, rather than damage it;
- terms and conditions of work that match business need with the desires and priorities of people in the *middle* stages of life.

There is great potential for development in this area. Ill health is the most common cause of early retirement. Yet, work in appropriate circumstances is also one of the strongest promoters of good health. Those who extend their working life tend to live longer.

Conclusion

So, if innovative action is taken in the next few years we could see:

- at least a million more people over 50 in work in the UK, many of whom will be over state pension age;

- a decline in the use of fixed retirement ages by employers, so that in practice when we retire is a matter of mutual agreement between employer and employee (as it already is for many);
- a spread of flexible pathways from main career to full retirement with gradual transitions in ways that will benefit both employer and employee;
- a reduction in the wide gulf between those with resources, choice and capacity to manage decisions on work and retirement and those who have none of these and no personal control over the course of events.
- the declining significance of state pension age as a single point defining the end of working life, and beginning of retirement as choice about when people take the state pension becomes common;
- a secure and stable settlement of state and private pension systems that is comprehensible to the public and gives a clear incentive to save rather than spend everything now;
- many more businesses where the age profile of the workforce more closely matches the age profile of its customers;
- a modest flow of employment tribunal cases about age discrimination because the great majority of organizations will respond to the new legislative framework and legal action will be the last resort;
- a sea change in the culture of advice, debate, and choice on midlife career change;
- a great expansion of opportunities in the workplace and in government programmes to train in flexible ways, either to return to a former occupation or start a new one.

Bibliography

Beveridge, W. (1942) *Social Insurance and Allied Services*, the Beveridge Report. London: Her Majesty's Stationery Office.

CBI (2004) *Official Response to Pensions Green Paper, Simplicity, Security and choice: Working and Saving for Retirement.* London: Confederation of British Industry. (www.cbi.org.uk/ndbs/positiondoc.nsf).

CEHR (2008) *Commission on Equality and Human Rights*, London (www.equalityhumanrights.com).

Daniel Dorling, D., Jan Rigby, J., Wheeler, B., Ballas, D., Thomas, B., Fahmy, E., Gordon, D. and Lupton, R. (2007) *Poverty, Wealth and Place in Britain 1968 to 2005.* York: Joseph Rowntree Foundation (www.jrf.org.uk).

DEE (1999) *Age Diversity in Employment: Encouraging Age Diversity. A Code of Practice.* London: Department of Education and Employment.

DEE (1988) *Code of Good Practice on the Employment of Disabled People*. London: Department of Employment.

DWP (2004) *The Pension Commission First Report,* October. London: Department of Work and Pensions.

DWP (2005) *Opportunity Age: A Strategy for an Ageing Society*. London: Department of Work and Pensions (www.dwp.gov.uk/opportunity_age/).

DWP (2008) *Good Practice in Employment*. London: Department of Work and Pensions (www.agepositive.gov.uk).

DWP (2008) Department of Work and Pensions, London (www.jobcentreplus.gov.uk/JCP/Customers).

DWP and DIUS (2007) *Opportunity, Employment, Progression: Making Skills Work*. Department of Work and Pensions and Department of Innovation, Universities and Skills (www.dwp.gov.uk/welfarereform).

EFA (2008) *Good Practice on Age Diversity*. London: The Employers Forum on Age (www.efa.org.uk).

ELMR (2007) *Economic & Labour Market Review*. Basingstoke: Palgrave Macmillan.

HMSO (2006) *The Employment Equality (Age) Regulations 2006,* Statutory Instrument 2006, No. 1031 Her Majesty's Stationery Office (www.opsi.gov.uk).

HMT (2006) *Prosperity for All in the Global Economy – World Class Skills,* the Leitch Review, London: Her Majesty's Treasury (www.hm treasury.gov.uk/independent_reviews/leitch_review).

ONS (2006) *Annual Survey of Hours and Earnings*. London: Office of National Statistics (www.statistics.gov.uk).

Ray, S., Sharp, E. and Abrams, D. (2005) *Ageism: A Benchmark of Public Attitudes in Britain*. Canterbury: University of Kent for Age Concern (www.ageconcern.org.uk/AgeConcern/Documents/Ageism_Report).

TAEN (2006) *Facts and Figures on Pensions and Retirement*. London: The Age and Employment Network (www.taen.org.uk/resources).

TAEN (2007a) *Managing the Ageing Workforce: An Introductory Guide to Age Management for HR Professionals*. London: The Age and Employment Network (www.taen.org.uk).

TAEN (2007b) *Key Facts on Health, Age and Employment*. London: The Age and Employment Network (www.taen.org.uk/resources).

8 Changing life course transitions: implications for work and lifelong learning

Chris Phillipson

Introduction

For much of its brief history, research in the field of ageing has been influenced by a particular view concerning the shape of the life course. In general terms, the period from 1945 to the mid-1970s was influenced by the idea of a 'standardized' life course built around what was described as the 'three boxes' of education, work and leisure (Best 1980). In the case of Western industrial societies (and mainly in the case of men in contrast to women), this phase came to be associated with the creation of the institution of retirement together with gradual acceptance of an extended period of leisure following the ending of full-time work (Phillipson 1998).

From the mid-1970s, a number of changes can be discerned arising from the development of more flexible patterns of work and the impact of globalization on patterns of employment. These produced what came to be termed the reconstruction of middle and old age, with the identification of a 'third age' in between the period of work and employment ('the second age') and that of a period of mental and physical decline ('the fourth age'). A characteristic feature of this new period of life is the ambiguity and flexibility of its boundaries at the lower and upper ends (Moen 2003). Both are seen to involve complex periods of transition, with greater ambiguity associated with the move away from employment, and with the blurring of dependence and independence with physical and mental deterioration (see also Dannefer 2002).

These changes have set a comprehensive research agenda for gerontology, as well as having a substantial impact on the lives of men and women entering their 50s. This chapter is divided into four sections: first, some general issues associated with the changes in midlife transitions are reviewed;

second, the implications of these for the organization of work are assessed; third, responses in the areas of education and training are considered; fourth, the chapter reviews a key policy option for future development.

Changing work and retirement transitions

In recent years, issues relating to older workers and retirement have become major influences affecting the development of economic and social policy (Nyce and Schieber 2005; Reday-Mulvay 2005). In part, this has reflected significant changes to retirement as a social institution. Donald Hirsch (2003) has observed that through the twentieth century, the idea of a fixed point of leaving work – at 60 or 65 – developed as one of the great certainties of life, most especially in the case of men. Modern retirement policy was itself a product of the late nineteenth century, as large private companies and branches of the civil service adopted pension policies of different kinds. Subsequently, at key periods in the twentieth century (e.g. periods of economic depression) pension provision was extended to a wider range of groups (Hannah 1986; Meadows 2003; Macnicol 1998). In consequence, modern states became responsible not only for the income maintenance of substantial sections of the older population but also for determining the rules governing access to different pathways into retirement (Kohli et al. 1991).

Over the past 10 years these 'pathways' or 'transitions' have become more diverse than was previously the case. Donald Hirsch has summarized some of the changes as follows:

- Fewer than four in ten men are still working immediately before reaching the state pension age (compared with six out of ten in 1980).
- Of people leaving full-time permanent jobs between 50 and state pension age (SPA), nearly as many enter part-time, temporary or self-employed work as stop working immediately.
- While men (to a greater extent than women) are much more likely to leave work before SPA than a generation ago, the UK government wants to encourage more to continue after this age, by improving incentives to defer the state pension.
- Ensuring adequate income in later life has become a complex process, with greater responsibility falling to individuals than in the initial Beveridge system. The structure of pensions is more diverse with the basic state pension joined by an array of means-tested credits, second state pensions, personal pensions and occupational pensions.

(Hirsch 2003: 7)

Changes to retirement as an institution have, then, been one element driving a number of discussions within economic and social policy. Underpinning these, however, has been a generalized concern regarding employment issues in relation to older workers (Phillipson and Smith 2005). Employment rates for men aged 50–SPA have fallen dramatically since the mid-1970s, albeit with some recovery since the late-1990s and with noticeable increases in rates for women. This development, while accepted (and indeed in part promoted by government policy) over the course of the 1980s and early 1990s, came under scrutiny from the late-1990s onwards. Governmental and non-governmental agencies put the case for limiting the withdrawal of people 50 and over from the workplace, and encouraging those economically inactive back into work (Department for Work and Pensions (DWP) 2005; Robinson et al. 2005).

The focus on older workers arose in part from concerns around age discrimination in the workplace (Macnicol 2006), illustrated in the DWP *Age Positive Campaign* and their *Code of Practice on Age Diversity in Employment.* Wider influences were, however, present; these including, first, labour market pressures associated with the likely increase in numbers of older people in the workplace (projections indicating around 32 per cent of the working-age population aged 50 and over by 2021); second, developments in the field of pensions, including modifications to occupational pension rules, which aimed at extending working life and encouraging greater flexibility in options about when to retire; third, concern over the desirability of early retirement, with the social and personal costs emphasized in documents such as *Winning the Generation Game* (Performance and Innovation Unit (PIU) 2000) and *Opportunity Age* (DWP 2005).

The policy of extending working lives has been a significant outcome of the debate concerning the economic sustainability of ageing populations, reflected in large measure by the above concerns. In essence, the discussion has shifted from focusing upon *early retirement/early exit* to identifying *pathways into work,* with particular encouragement given to work beyond SPA. The aim is to reverse the trend – characteristic of the 1980s and 1990s – whereby large numbers of older workers left work ahead of SPA, and where early retirement came to be accepted as a normal event in the life course (Marshall et al. 2001).

The extent of the decline in employment among older workers is important to acknowledge, especially given policy ambitions of removing barriers to employment. The dominant pattern, stretching over nearly three decades, has been a declining age of exit from the labour force – a trend that accelerated over the course of the 1970s and 1980s (Laczko and Phillipson 1991). Even up to 1971, 93 per cent of men in Britain aged 55–59 and 83 per cent aged 60–64 were economically active, with around 19 per cent of men working on after SPA. The highest figure recorded was in 1961 when labour force participation rates reached 97 per cent among men aged 55–59 and 91 per cent for those aged 60–64. By 1989, however, the rate for men aged 55–59 had dropped to 79.8 per cent and for those 60–64 to 54.6 per cent. In other words, while in 1950 the average age of exit (for men) from employment was 67.2 years, with 18 years spent in retirement, by 1990 the average age had dropped to 63.5 per cent with 27 years now spent in the period following cessation of work (Pensions Commission 2004).

Over the course of the 1990s, with the move out of economic recession, the pattern of early exit from work went into reverse with increases in economic activity for men and women in their 50s and 60s (Organization for Economic Cooperation and Development (OECD) 2006). This trend has continued into the opening decade of the twenty-first century: the Labour Force Survey (LFS) for Great Britain shows a rise in employment for men aged 50–SPA from 68.7 per cent in 1999 to 72.8 per cent in 2007; equivalent figures for women increasing from 63.4 per cent to 70.1 per cent. There were also increases over the same period for those over SPA: among men, from 7.6 per cent to 9.9 per cent; for women, from 8.1 per cent to 11.7 per cent.

The Pensions Commission (2004: 38; see also Hotopp 2005) identified the upward move in employment rates among those 50–SPA as the result of four main effects:

1. *Demand side factors* such as the absence of major macro-economic shocks comparable to the 1970s/1980s; this producing fewer redundancies and the possibility of re-entry into the labour market once unemployed.
2. *Supply-side factors* such as changes in pensions, in particular with the move, first, from *'defined benefit'* (DB) to *'defined contribution'* (DC) schemes – retirement behaviour in the latter tending towards later retirement given the context of a fall in equity markets and a reduction in annuities. Second, reduced opportunities for early retirement on grounds of 'ill health' as a result of tax penalties on early retirement 'packages' in the private sector and a range of restrictions on retirement ahead of SPA in the public sector.
3. Pressures arising from the substantial deficits that had developed in many company pension funds.
4. Closure or restriction of pathways into early retirement (e.g. changes in eligibility tests for disability benefits; initiatives to encourage disability beneficiaries back into the workplace).

Phillipson (2004) noted an additional factor in the encouragement of gradual pathways to retirement, such as part-time work and self-employment (18 per cent of those 50–SPA are self-employed compared with 12 per cent of 25–49-year-olds and 4 per cent of 16–24-year-olds). Such 'bridging' forms of employment have become increasingly significant for men as well as women in managing transitions from work to retirement (Phillipson 2002; Platman 2004; Loretto et al. 2005; see further discussion below). The development of programmes such as New Deal 50 plus in encouraging training and returning to work may have had some influence, although Disney and Hawkes (2003: 67) argue that this may be: '... through their symbolic importance and the association with relatively favourable demand conditions, rather than through the measures themselves'.

Despite the upward move in employment rates, most people once reaching SPA (nearly 90 per cent according to the LFS) become classified as 'economically inactive'; and this still applies to around one in four of those 50–SPA (with ill health or sickness a major factor). Moreover, all the 50+ age group are affected by the evolution of the more complex transitions associated with what Giddens (1991) has defined as a post-industrial life course. Here, the evidence suggests that the apparent stability of work-retirement transitions in the 1950s and 1960s (limited in any event to men in secure occupations) was almost certainly a brief interlude in what has always been an unsettled period of the life course. What came to be seen as the norm in this period was the idea of a 'crisp' transition from employment to retirement at a standard age (e.g. 60 or 65). Increasingly, however, departure from work is 'blurred' rather than 'crisp' and may involve a number of moves in and out of paid work (Marshall et al. 2001; Phillipson 2002; Vickerstaff 2006).

Moen (2003) identifies an emerging life stage between the years of career-building and old age, a period stretching roughly from age 50 to age 75. She sees this new phase as creating a mixture of uncertainties and opportunities: the former reflected in pressures and insecurities in the workplace (with downsizing and forced early retirement); the latter developed through a broadening in the range of productive activities (with combinations of work, caring and leisure activities).

A further influence, resulting in the 'loosening' of life course boundaries, has been the collapse of the work-based bureaucracies associated with what Richard Sennett (2006) refers to as 'social capitalism'. This form of capitalism had at its centre the rationalized organization of time that framed work careers (notably for men) as long term and incremental:

> Rationalized time enabled people to think about their lives as narratives – narratives not so much of what necessarily will happen as of how things should happen. It became possible, for instance, to define what the stages of a career ought to be like, to correlate long-term service in a firm to specific steps of increased wealth.
>
> (Sennett 2006: 23)

Sennett's (2006: 183) main point is that the erosion of social capitalism has 'deprived people of [this] sense of *narrative movement*' (author's emphasis).

Elsewhere, he sets out a number of important questions that he sees as following from this development, namely: 'How can long-term purposes be pursued in a short-term society? How can durable social relationships be sustained? How can a human being develop a narrative of identity and life history in a society composed of episodes and fragments?' (Sennett 1999: 26).

In terms of the work-retirement transition, a number of empirical findings illustrate this 'disruption' in narrative movement. The emergence of so-called 'bridge jobs', along with the rise of self-employment, might be cited as one example, such employment becoming increasingly common for women and men in their 50s and 60s in the UK and the USA. Cahill et al.'s (2006: 523) research using data from the *US Health and Retirement Study* found that the majority of older Americans leaving full-time career employment (about 60 per cent of those leaving a full-time career job after 50 and about 53 per cent of those leaving after the age of 55) moved first to a bridge job rather than directly out of the labour force. Analysis of the *British Household Panel Survey*, examining job movements among men in their 50s, indicated around one in five had spells of part-time, bridging forms of employment (Phillipson 2002).

On the one hand, such movements might, from one perspective, be taken as illustrative of the emergence of greater choice for individuals in reshaping the ending of their work careers. On the other hand, the reality, however, suggests otherwise, with many moving into 'bridge employment' out of 'financial necessity' and often into contingent or 'non-core' areas of the workforce (Phillipson 2002; Cahill et al. 2006). Cahill et al. comment here that:

> Bridge jobs can provide older [workers] with the opportunity to stay active and productive, to experience a different line of work, and to earn income ... For others, however, especially those at the lower end of the socio-economic scale, bridge jobs may reflect financial necessity – an unfortunate and undesirable finale during the twilight of their work career.
>
> (Cahill et al. 2006: 523)

Narrative movement or continuity may be further frustrated by high levels of stress within the workplace, evidence for which has again been reported in UK as well as US data. Among white-collar employees, the role of stress in the workplace may be an important factor precipitating withdrawal from work. In a UK longitudinal study of early retirement, Higgs et al. report that:

> when health problems were mentioned, they were generally described in terms of stress ... [they go to note that] it is possible that these results reflect a new pattern of early retirement in which

> mental health as well as economic considerations feature in the early retirement decisions among white collar workers.
>
> (Higgs et al. 2008: 771)

More general problems associated with work may also 'push' people out of the labour market. Green (2005) has reviewed a number of large data sets which suggest significant declines in job satisfaction over the course of the 1990s. The programme of research on *Transitions to Retirement* conducted by the Joseph Rowntree Foundation (e.g. Barnes et al. 2002; Hirsch 2005) found that many people leaving work early disliked their jobs because they felt they were not leading anywhere; they also felt themselves to be undervalued by their employers (Hirsch 2005). In the UK survey by Humphrey et al. (2003), 31 per cent of men gave a work-related reason for their early retirement; 37 per cent in the case of women. Eleven per cent of men and 16 per cent of women reported that their work had become too 'physically demanding'; 8 per cent of both reported that it had become too stressful. Such findings are reflected in the extent of 'under-employment' or 'semi-employment' affecting a substantial group of older workers – around one-fifth of men in their 50s according to one estimate for the USA (Sennett 2006).

One general implication of the above concerns the extent to which the life course for many has been reconstructed, but on terms over which individuals have limited control (Vickerstaff and Cox 2005). E.P. Thompson (1967) in his essay 'Time, work-discipline and industrial capitalism' suggested that: '... mature industrial societies of all varieties [are] marked by a clear demarcation between "work" and "life".' He went on to put the following question in his essay: '... if Puritanism was a necessary part of the work-ethos which enabled the industrialized world to break out of the poverty-stricken economies of the past, will the Puritan valuation of time begin to decompose as the pressures of poverty relax ...Will men begin to lose that restless urgency, that desire to consume purposively, which most people carry just as they carry the watch on their wrist?'

For a period, when the 'golden age' of capitalism (Glyn 2006) had reached its full maturity, the possibility of a 'third age' characterized by free time appeared to be on the horizon (Laslett 1989). True, its appearance was stronger for men in full-time employment than women (who remained in mainly poorly-paid part-time employment combined with intensive caring and domestic roles); and was certainly much less relevant to the lives of many minority ethnic groups and migrant workers (as indeed remains the case). But the changes with social capitalism have introduced new pressures and inequalities for the majority of those moving through work into retirement. In the words of Richard Sennett (1999: 146): 'Who needs me?' is a question of character which suffers a radical challenge in modern capitalism. The system radiates indifference. It does so in terms of the outcomes of human striving, as in winner-take-all markets, where there is little connection between risk and reward. It radiates indifference in the organization of absence of trust, where there is no reason to be needed. And it does so through re-engineering of institutions in which people are treated as disposable. Such practices obviously and brutally diminish the sense of mattering as a person, of being necessary to others.

Finding reasons to *'matter to others'* (to paraphrase Sennett) is fundamental to securing a viable transition in the move from work to retirement. Gerontology has embraced this issue through the work of Achenbaum (2005) and others, in calling for a 'wider vision' of later-life productivity, embracing themes such as altruism, citizenship, stewardship and creativity. Yet this call will struggle for realization given the disruption of narratives around work and those in related areas such as pensions (Blackburn 2007). One possibility here, however, is that workplace training and education could be used to develop and extend skills to support people both in work and in the move into retirement. The next section considers evidence about the influence of activity in this area, assessing the evidence for support for older workers in work-based training.

Training and education in the work and retirement transition

The benefits of learning and training, across all age groups, are now widely acknowledged. The Department for Education and Skills (2005) argues that there is good evidence that 'older people can benefit substantially from continuing to learn and gain new skills' (para. 210). Given a policy of extending the period of employment, the expectation must be that older workers will have an equal opportunity with younger age groups of sharing in different types of training and learning. In reality, younger adults are better qualified than older adults. In 2004, 79 per cent of 25–29-year-olds were qualified to level 2 or higher compared to 67 per cent of adults aged over 50. In recent years there has been more improvement among younger adults than older adults and so the gap has widened from nearly 8 percentage points in 1997 to nearly 13 percentage points in 2004 (DES 2005).

Evidence from a variety of data sources suggests that older workers continue to be disadvantaged in respect of training received while employed. Stoney and Roberts's (2003) analysis of data from the 2002 LFS indicated that workers aged 50 and over were 50 per cent less likely than their younger colleagues to receive on- or off-the-job training. Further analysis of the LFS by Newton et al. (2005) found that employees working in 'unskilled occupations' were the least likely to receive training, with as few as 7 per cent of 60–64-year-olds in elementary occupations engaged in training (see also Humphreys et al. 2003; Urwin 2004).

Such findings are supported by Humphrey et al. (2003) who found that while most employees received some encouragement to learn more job-related skills, this tended to tail off after age 50–54. Thus, among men, 58 per cent in this age group had received a great deal or a fair amount of encouragement; this compared with 42 per cent for those aged 55–59 and 41 per cent for those aged 60–64. Among women, the equivalent figures for the 50–54 and 60–64 age groups were 63 per cent and 40 per cent.

Lissenburgh and Smeaton's (2003) analysis of LFS data confirmed the link between increased age and declining access to training. Logistic regression models used in their study also suggested that men and women in part-time and temporary employment were especially disadvantaged in respect of training. Humphreys et al. (2003) also found that the level of encouragement to undertake training varied between full- and part-time employees. In their survey one-third of part-time employees were offered no encouragement to learn more job-related skills, compared with one-quarter of full-time employees. These findings were confirmed by Arulampalam et al. (2003) using data from the *European Community Household Panel* (ECHP). This study investigated gender differences in training participation over the period 1994–1999, with particular attention to type of employment contract and sector affiliation. The research found that for men, being on a fixed-term contract was associated with a significantly lower probability of training. Employees in the UK on part-time contracts were in general less likely to receive training than their counterparts in other European countries. Comparative data also shows the UK performing well below the Organization for Economic Cooperation and Development (OECD) average for expected hours in non-formal job-related education and training (OECD 2007).

More information is required about the degree to which older workers themselves fail to take up opportunities for education and training. This may happen where they lack confidence about learning new skills (Newton et al. 2003) or because they feel that acquiring them is no longer necessary or may go unrewarded (McNair 2005). Taylor and Urwin's (2001) research conducted in the late 1990s suggested that declining participation in training was linked to employer decision-making rather than an individual preference not to undertake training. Urwin (2004: 28), on the other hand, argues that there is some evidence to suggest that not only is training less likely to be offered to older individuals, but also that 'large proportions of this group have not taken up the opportunity to train'. Moss and Arrowsmith (2003: 24) concur with this suggesting that 'attitudinal barriers' can limit responses to training: '... some [Jobcentre] customers may either feel that it is too late in their life to learn basic skills that they have managed to survive without for so long, or, if they have worked before, that they do not need a course that offers basic employability skills'. The evaluation of New Deal 50 plus also questioned the intrinsic value placed on training by older workers. Atkinson

(2003) provided evidence to suggest that in some cases older people were overskilled for their current job and therefore do not see training as relevant.

Employers are likely to vary considerably in their approach to training. McNair et al. (2004) found that people in large firms continued to develop skills in a way that was less true of those in small- and medium-sized enterprises (SMEs). Some occupational sectors (notably managerial and professional groups) appear much more likely to support training than others (e.g. those in elementary occupations). And level of skill and qualification (or human capital) appears critical – those with higher degrees and/or professional qualifications are more likely to participate in training later in working life compared with those with lower-level qualifications (Newton et al. 2003). For professional/managerial groups, external pressure to extend working life may not be a major issue given that higher qualifications and socio-economic class are strong predictors of longer working life (McNair 2005). For some manual groups, deficits in training over the life course may be difficult to correct, especially given limited workplace opportunities and depressed expectations about learning.

Gender may play a significant role in gaining access to training. Taylor and Urwin (2001) found that men aged 50–64 were 2 per cent less likely to have been offered training and 12.3 per cent less likely to have received training in the last 13 weeks, relative to the reference group of prime-age individuals (aged 25–39). For women, the effects were much smaller, with females over 50 to retirement age 5.5 per cent less likely to undergo training when compared with their prime-age counterparts.

Newton et al. (2005) reviewed the availability of training among those unemployed and economically inactive. This study shows that overall less than one in ten report involvement in training and that training participation declines rapidly with age. The likelihood of someone aged 55 and over participating in training is 50 per cent less compared with an adult aged 35–44. McNair et al. (2004) found that levels of support given to those changing their job declined with age. Older workers were less likely than younger ones to receive any help during a job transition (37 per cent of older workers, against 47 per cent of those under 50). They were less likely to receive training from their employers; help from their workmates and colleagues; or support from a government agency. They were also less likely to have sort out support from themselves, either through the Internet or other informal sources.

To the above, largely negative findings, must be balanced more positive developments which may be important over the medium and longer term. Future generations of older workers can be expected to have higher levels of basic numeracy and literacy skills and this should have a major impact on areas such as participation in continuing education and training. Dixon (2003: 74) notes from the LFS the strong relationship between level of qualification and the likelihood of undertaking job-related training, as well as the finding that those with higher existing qualifications are more likely to be studying for a new qualification. She concludes that these relationships suggest that age-specific differentials in learning activity could flatten in future as the fraction of older workers who have not completed secondary education gradually declines.

There is also evidence that older people are just as willing to invest in learning new skills as younger age groups. Taylor and Urwin (2001: 769) found that despite the shorter time horizons of those in the 50–59/64 age group, a similar proportion to those in the 25–39 and 40–40 age groups (20 per cent) had self-financed their own training. Sustained economic growth should also have some impact in reducing training differentials between age groups. Urwin (2004: 29) suggests some 'catch up' in the period over 1992 and 2002 when comparing the training received by older and younger workers; this reflecting a cyclical component with improved economic prospects allowing firms to increase the amount of money allotted to formal education and training.

Developing education policies for the work-retirement transition

The extent of change running through the period of midlife from the 50s onwards suggests the need for innovation in key areas of public policy. Among these, access to training and education in the second half of the life course will be a crucial area for development. Ford (2005a) makes the point that although many adults 50–SPA have highly developed skills and experience currently lost to the economy, learning requirements are higher than for younger age groups. He notes that one in three in this group have literacy or numeracy problems, compared with one in five of those aged 26–35. Mayhew and Rijkers (2004) stress the importance of 'continuous learning during the whole of working life as a means of reducing the dangers of labour market disadvantage in the older years'. Ford (2005b: 10) makes the case for an 'overall national third age guidance and learning strategy, one which would be linked to the national skills strategy and which would enable adults from midlife onwards to maximize their skills and potential'. Assisting this will, however, require a reversal of current policies which are reducing public funding for adult learners. Aldridge and Tuckett highlight this point as follows:

> ... since 2005 a million adult learners have been lost to publicly funded adult learning and the greatest loss has been suffered by learners over 65 where numbers in 2006–07 are less than half the

> 2004–05 totals in further education, and 30 per cent lower in what the government call 'personal and community development learning'. These changes will inevitably impact on participation overall – however much older people fund organised and self-funded alternatives.
>
> (Aldridge and Tuckett 2007: 5)

An important element in any strategy must be closer involvement from higher education and further education institutions in responding to the needs of older learners, with the development of new programmes or the adaptation of existing ones to the needs of 'third age employees'. Older students have always had an important presence in university adult education classes, with those aged over 50 comprising the majority of participants. They also form a significant group in part-time degrees and courses in continuing professional development. Some 39 per cent of all students study part time; 90 per cent of part-time undergraduate students are over 21, with around 20 per cent in their 40s and 15 per cent now aged over 50.

At present, higher education has made only limited responses to the impact of demographic change. There is growing realization of the consequences arising from a decline in young school leavers, the group who have formed the great majority of full-time higher education entrants. Although numbers among this group will increase up to 2010–11, there are likely to be significant reductions thereafter (Bekhradnia 2007). A number of policies are available for reducing the impact of demographic change, not least increasing participation rates among young people from working-class backgrounds, and increasing provision for flexible study (notably courses which can be studied on a part-time basis). However, increasing the level of engagement among people aged 50+ in higher education and further education colleges will also be of considerable importance. For this to happen, however, higher education will need to actively embrace older people as a major group in future educational programmes. Consideration will need to be given to the type of curricula relevant to different groups within the 50+ population; the range of learning styles that need to be catered for, and the changes generated by new cohorts with higher levels of educational attainment. In responding to these issues, the call made by Harry Moody remains highly relevant:

> ... education can contribute dramatically to quality of life in old age. To make a case for a wider public policy supporting late-life education, we need to see quality of life issues in a broader context ... public policy ... still looks on education of old people as a frill, as inessential, strictly as a matter of private decisions, and, above all, as something that does not cost any money and certainly is not worth spending any money on. How would we feel if health care or the

> education of children were seen in that way? We need to take late life education with more seriousness instead of seeing it as a way of filling up time for the old folks ... The potential for lifespan development through education is clear. But what remains unclear is whether our major social institutions will move toward providing those opportunities in the years to come.
>
> (Moody 1988: 212)

Achieving this, however, will require reversing the current situation, which sees participation in adult education and training falling precisely at the point (when people are in their 40s) when this area could play an influential role in helping people 'step up' into new roles and activities. This decline is a feature of virtually all industrialized countries, with Finland, Sweden and Norway notable exceptions. Platman (1999, 2004) points to the 'cycle of deskilling' affecting older workers, as a result of limited educational opportunities and restricted job-relating training. The consequences of such 'deskilling' may spill over into other areas relevant to life after age 50 and create problems in how individuals adjust to the various transitions running through the second half of the life course.

Conclusion

This chapter has highlighted the need to redefine the scope of midlife, given the major changes affecting the traditional life course. The challenge for social policy is to create the conditions for greater choice within the transitions encountered after age 50. This needs to be done in ways that maximize social inclusion in respect of more flexible lifestyles characteristic of life in the twenty-first century. The danger is that inaction will lead to large numbers of people experiencing new forms of insecurity given the transformation in the institutions of work and retirement. Life after age 50 appears to be a problem because of the apparent lack of substance to the roles that supersede or run alongside those associated with paid employment. Conducting a debate about the future of these roles will be an essential starting point for resolving dilemmas in a crucial area for economic and social policy.

References

Achenbaum, W.A. (2005) *Older Americans, Vital Communities*. Baltimore MD: John Hopkins Press.

Aldridge, F. and Tuckett, A. (2007) *What Older People Learn*. Leicester: National Institute for Adult and Continuing Education.

Arulampalam, W., Booth, A. and Bryn, M. (2003) *Training in Europe*, Institute for Social and Economic Research (ISER), Working Papers No. 2003–23, Colchester, University of Essex, ISER.

Atkinson, J. (2003) *Evaluation of the New Deal 50-plus: Summary Report.* Brighton: The Institute for Employment Studies.

Barnes, H., Parry, J. and Lakey, J. (2002) *Forging a New Future: The Experiences and Expectations of People Leaving Paid Work Over 50.* Bristol: The Policy Press.

Bekhradnia, B. (2007) *Demand for Higher Education to 2020 and Beyond.* London: Higher Education Policy Institute.

Best, F. (1980) *Flexible Life Scheduling.* New York: Praeger.

Blackburn, R. (2007) *Age Shock.* London: Verso.

Cahill, K., Giandrea, M. and Quinn, J. (2006) Retirement patterns from career employment, *The Gerontologist,* 46(4): 514–23.

Dannefer, D. (2002) Whose life course is it anyway? Diversity and 'linked lives' in global perspective, in R. Settersten (ed.) *Invitation to the Life Course.* Amityville, NY: Baywood.

Department for Education and Skills (DfES) (2005) *Skills: Getting On in Business, Getting On at Work,* Parts 1–3. London: The Stationery Office (TSO).

Department for Work and Pensions (DWP) (2005) *Opportunity Age.* London: Her Majesty's Stationery Office (HMSO).

Disney, R. and Hawkes, D. (2003) Why has employment recently risen among older workers, in R. Dickens, P. Gregg and J. Wadsworth (eds) *The Labour Market Under New Labour.* Basingstoke: Palgrave.

Dixon, S. (2003) Implications of population ageing for the labour market, *Labour Market Trends,* February: 67–76.

Ford, G. (2005a) *Am I Still Needed? Guidance and Learning for Older Adults.* Derby: The University of Derby, Centre for Guidance Studies.

Ford, G. (2005b) Am I still needed? Guidance and learning for older adults, Summary of Report, in D. Hirsch (ed.) *Sustaining Working Lives: A Framework for Policy and Practice.* York: Joseph Rowntree Foundation.

Giddens, A. (1991) *Modernity and Self-identity.* Cambridge: Polity Press.

Glyn, A. (2006) *Capitalism Unleashed.* Oxford: Oxford University Press.

Green, F. (2005) *Understanding Trends in Job Satisfaction: Final Report,* Report to the ESRC. Swindon: Economic and Social Research Council.

Hannah, L. (1986) *Inventing Retirement.* Cambridge: Cambridge University Press.

Higgs, P., Mein, G., Ferrie, J., Hyde, M. and Nazroo, J. (2003) Pathways to early retirement: structure and agency in decision-making among British civil servants, *Ageing and Society*, 23: 761–78.

Hirsch, D. (2003) Crossroads after 50: improving choices in work and retirement, *Foundations*, York: Joseph Rowntree Foundation.

Hirsch, D. (2005) *Sustaining Working Lives: A Framework for Policy and Practice.* York: Joseph Rowntree Foundation.

Hotopp, U. (2005) The employment rate of older workers, *Labour Market Trends*, 113: 73–86.

Humphrey, A., Costigan, P., Pickering, K., Stratford, N. and Barnes, M. (2003) *Factors Affecting the Labour Market: Participation of Older Workers*. London: Department of Work and Pensions.

Kohli, M., Rein, M., Guillemard, A-M. and van Gunsteren, H. (1991) *Time for Retirement: Comparative Studies of Early Exit from the Labour Force*. Cambridge: Cambridge University Press.

Laczko, F. and Phillipson, C. (1991) *Changing Work and Retirement.* Milton Keynes: Open University Press.

Laslett, P. (1989) *A Fresh Map of Life*. Cambridge: Cambridge University Press.

Lissenburgh, S. and Smeaton, D. (2003) *Employment Transitions of Older Workers: The Role of Flexible Employment in Maintaining Labour Market Participation and Promoting Job Quality*. Bristol/York: The Policy Press/Joseph Rowntree Foundation.

Loretto, W., Vickerstaff, S. and White, P. (2005) Older workers and options for flexible work, *Working Paper No. 31*, Manchester: Equal Opportunities Commission.

Macnicol, J. (1998) *The Politics of Retirement in Britain, 1878–1948*. Cambridge: Cambridge University Press.

Macnicol, J. (2006) *Age Discrimination*. Cambridge: Cambridge University Press.

Marshall, V.W., Heinz, W.R., Kűger, H. and Vermer, A. (eds) (2001) *Restructuring Work and the Life Course*. Toronto: University of Toronto Press.

Mayhew, K. and Rijkers, B. (2004) How to improve the human capital of older workers, or the sad tail of the magic bullet, Paper prepared for the joint EC OECD seminar on Human Capital and Labour Market Performance, Brussels, 8 December.

McNair, S. (2005) The age of choice: a new agenda for learning and work, in A. Tuckett and A. McAulay (eds) *Demography and Older Learners*, pp. 27–38. Leicester: National Institute of Adult Continuing Education (NIACE).

McNair, S., Flynn, M., Owen, L., Humphreys, C. and Woodfield, S. (2004) *Changing Work in Later Life: A Study of Job Transitions*. Guildford: University of Surrey, Centre for Research into the Older Workforce.

Meadows, P. (2003) *Retirement Ages in the UK: A Review of the Literature*, Employment Relations Research Series No. 18. London: Department of Trade and Industry.

Moen, P. (2003) Midcourse: reconfiguring careers and community service for a new life stage, *Contemporary Gerontology*, 9: 87–94.

Moody, H. (1988) *Abundance of Life: Human Development Policies for an Aging Society*. New York: Columbia University Press.

Moss, N. and Arrowsmith, J. (2003) *A Review of What Works for Clients Over 50*. Sheffield: Department for Work and Pensions.

Newton, B., Hurstfield, J., Miller, L., Ackroyd, K. and Gifford, J. (2003) *Training Participation Amongst Unemployed and Inactive People*. Brighton: Institute for Employment Studies.

Newton, B., Hurstfield, J., Miller, L. and Bates, P. (2005) *Training a Mixed Age Workforce: Practical Tips and Guidance*. London: Department of Work and Pensions.

Nyce, S. and Schieber, S. (2005) *The Economic Implication of Aging Societies*. Cambridge: Cambridge University Press.

Organization for Economic Cooperation and Development (OECD) (2006) *Live Longer, Work Longer*. Paris: OECD.

Organization for Economic Cooperation and Development (OECD) (2007) *Education at a Glance*. Paris: OECD.

Pensions Commission (2004) *Pensions: Challenges and Choices*. Norwich: The First Report of the Pensions Commission, The Stationery Office (TSO).

Phillipson, C. (1998) *Reconstructing Old Age*. London: Sage Publications.

Phillipson, C. (2002) *Transitions from Work to Retirement: Developing a New Social Contract*. Bristol/York: The Policy Press/Joseph Rowntree Foundation.

Phillipson, C. (2004) Work and retirement transitions: changing sociological and social policy contexts, *Social Policy and Society*, 3(2): 155–62.

Phillipson, C. and Smith, C. (2005) *Extending Working Life: A Review of the Research Literature*. London: Department of Work and Pensions.

Performance and Innovation Unit (PIU) (2000) *Winning the Generation Game.* London: The Stationery Office.

Platman, K. (1999) *The Glass Precipice: Employability for a Mixed Age Workforce.* London: Employers Forum on Ageing.

Platman, K. (2004) Flexible employment in later life: public policy panaceas in the search for mechanisms to extend working lives, *Social Policy and Society*, 3(2): 181–88.

Reday-Mulvay, G. (2005) *Working beyond 60: Key Policies and Practices in Europe.* London: Palgrave.

Robinson, P., Gosling, T. and Lewis, M. (2005) *Working Later: Raising the Effective Age of Retirement.* London: Institute for Public Policy Research (IPPR).

Sennett, R. (1999) *The Corrosion of Character.* New York: W.W.Norton.

Sennett, R. (2006) *The Culture of the New Capitalism.* New Haven, CT: Yale University Press.

Stoney, C. and Roberts, M. (2003) *The Case for Older Workers at Tesco: An Examination of Attitudes, Assumptions and Attributes,* Working Paper No. 53, Carlton University, School of Public Policy and Administration, Ottawa, Ontario.

Taylor, P. and Urwin, P. (2001) Age and participation in vocational education and training, *Work, Employment and Society*, 15: 763–79.

Thompson, E.P. (1967) Time, work-discipline and industrial capitalism, *Past and Present*, 36: 56–97.

Urwin, P. (2004) Age matters: a review of existing survey evidence, *Employment Relations Research Series No. 24.* London: Department of Trade and Industry.

Vickerstaff, S. (2006) Entering the retirement zone: how much choice do individuals have? *Social Policy and Society*, 5(4): 507–17.

Vickerstaff, S. and Cox, J. (2005) Retirement and risk: the individualisation of retirement and experiences? *The Sociological Review*, 53: 77–95.

9 Approaches to the 50+ workforce across Europe

Anthony Chiva with Philippe Gabriel, Grzegorz Karpiuk, Inés Dominguez López, Asmund Lunde, Yvan Paris, Adam Piekara, Jan Shepherd and Jorge Alonso Vallejo

This chapter reviews some approaches to working and managing the associated life changes among people aged 50 and over (50+). Other chapters in this book describe the situation for workers over 50 years old as being dynamic and complex, with many factors impacting on them. As the authors observe, many older workers are seeking to keep working longer (Centre for Research on the Older Worker 2004; Phillipson 2002; Worsley and Moynagh 2002). Therefore, when working with people aged 50+, approaches need to embrace a wide range of potential changes, including multiple routes into and out of work, education and leisure; a great variety of relationships patterns – changing partnerships and caring responsibilities; and more responsibility for personal finance and health. These changes provide both greater opportunity and greater risks on the later-life journey for older people (Beck 1998; Hirsh 2003). This chapter focuses on some exemplary European projects and ways of managing work and retirement: the 50+ Europe project (2002–2004), the Intergenerational Portfolio Management Project (2006–2008) and the Call to Action Project (Pension Education Fund 2007–2009).

The 50+ Europe project funded through the Leonardo da Vinci programme investigated approaches to 50+ employment and managing later-life changes in five countries (www.50pluseurope.co.uk). As with many other transnational projects, a range of European partners with diverse economic, political backgrounds and experiences of 50+ issues was involved: France, Norway, Poland, Spain and the United Kingdom (UK). These countries came together to explore ways of overcoming barriers to employing older people and ways of promoting age diversity with employers (Chiva et al. 2003).

The study found that European countries demonstrate a wide variety of political and economic perspectives for supporting 50+ workers. Those countries within the European Union (EU) have also been required to examine their labour policies by the EU directive on equality in employment (European Union 2006), which makes age discrimination illegal. The employment contexts in these countries were and still are highly variable, with different labour market conditions and priorities. The different countries involved in this project identified very different ways of encouraging employers and individuals to meet their employment needs.

However, one common thread among the participating countries is demographic transition, especially low fertility rates and an ageing population, which are facing most EU countries. This has led to shortages in and pressures on the labour market with subsequent raising of retirement ages, as a way to manage increasing social costs (pensions) and to address potential skills gaps. What was innovative in this project, however, was the focus of the partners in this project on highlighting the variety of approaches adopted by different European countries in the way they target particular age groups.

The age for targeting Inducements

In the pre-age legislation period when the 50+ Europe project was taking place, some countries (Norway, France and Spain) were seeking to use 'inducements' with employers, designed to encourage them to employ, retain and retrain older workers. These inducements or incentives came in two different forms:

1. financial benefits for employing older worker;
2. financial support for retraining older workers.

There were also penalties for economically active unemployed individuals who did not seek work.

Norway responded to labour shortages and a shrinking labour force over a number of years by focusing on 'senior policies' for people aged 60 years and over with government funding for a Centre for Senior Planning (2004). These 'senior policies' included the introduction of wage subsidies for employers, if they recruited long-term unemployed people over the age of 62. The Norwegian government also introduced flexible retirement, so that older workers could receive a partial pension while working and it gave entitlements to longer holidays for people continuing to work when aged over 60. This is comparable to later UK legislation on pensions (Department for Work and Pensions (DWP) 2006), which allows for the continuation of working after 65 years of age while being in receipt of state, personal and occupational pensions. These moves in the UK, as in Norway, are likely to impact on extending working lives. There are powerful economic drivers for people aged 55–65 to remain in work (McNair and Flynn 2005). The pressure to maintain income from paid work in order to supplement pensions and savings is also confirmed by UK government reports (DWP 2006). As can be seen, the target age here is not all older people but a particular segment.

In Spain and France, governments initiated financial contributions and tax incentives for employing older workers but at younger ages. In Spain the focus was on people who were long-term unemployed, aged over 40+ for women/45+ years for men (see Chapter 10 Making the most of experience – the East Midlands story which focuses on people aged 45+ years). These two countries also provided positive inducements to continue working and the potential withdrawal of some income-related benefits for not continuing in work, as in Norway for an older age group.

Enabling the individual to overcome barriers to employment

Systematic institutional ageism has been identified as a problem in many organizations and it has created difficulties for older individuals to continue employment into later life. Age legislation may only have a marginal impact on these barriers to employment (Taylor 2002; Walker 2005; Hagan Hennessy and Walker 2004; Phillipson 2004), as evidenced by the mixed effects of age legislation in other countries, such as the United States of America (USA).

The 50+ Europe project explored and recommended strategies to overcome barriers to employment for the over-50s. This challenge was tackled through two approaches: to employers in promoting the advantages of employing older workers, and through the over-50s themselves by supporting them in reviewing their options and in job-seeking and applications.

The project developed checklists for employers to support them in assessing their age diversity strategies and the extent to which they meet the European legislation of 2006 which makes age discrimination in employment illegal. These checklists built on the audit developed for employers in Norway by the Centre for Senior Planning – the Senior Planning Audit (2005c).

In each of the partner countries human resource (HR) managers and employers were consulted about their attitudes to employing older workers. Research reports and discussions with organizations with an interest in the over-50s in the workforce (in the UK these included the Chartered Institute for Personnel and Development, Third Age Employment Network, Employers Forum on Age, Help the Aged and Department of Work and Pensions) also informed the creation of the checklists. From workshops with HR staff it was possible to develop and gain feedback on the checklists during their development. For example, it emerged that separate checklists were needed for large and for small organizations as smaller companies or enterprises would not have dedicated HR departments, and often the company manager or owner would be responsible for recruitment and employment.

The 50+ Europe project developed and piloted materials, which enabled individuals aged 50+ to undertake a review of their work situation and to identify positive ways forward. The 50+ Workbook integrates theory with practice and provides structured activities, which supports people in assessing their own personalities and needs for paid employment. The materials were developed, designed and piloted within the project partnership of France, Poland, Norway, Spain and the UK, so that they have applicability across Europe.

The design process for the 50+ Workbook

The design of the materials for individuals was related to core principles and concepts about the ways that humans develop, create meaning in their lives and manage changes (Biggs 1999; Rogers 1986; Jung 1967; Coleman and Chiva 1992; Bridges 1995). The materials built on these core principles, extending them into the ways that people prioritize their lives (Covey et al. 1999). These were the starting points for the materials, and practical exercises were designed to enable the users, who were job-seekers, job changers and job retainers, to manage changes in their lives and employment around work.

From this base materials were developed jointly and then piloted in each partner country to test their effectiveness. In developing these materials, which have validity and application across a range of European partners, partners needed to take into consideration their different contexts: priorities for employment of different groups and which are most important to get into work; national socio-economic priorities and attitudes to social support; demographic profiles; skills gaps and shortages; and populations who have particular educational needs, preferences and styles with regard to activities/materials.

The process adopted to develop the 50+ materials was:

1 a transnational meeting to identify the key areas to be covered and issues in employment of people aged 50+;
2 establishment of national steering committees which included the key players and policy-makers in the support and employment of older people;

3. national research into the needs, priorities, training provision, support and employment of the 50+ population;
4. development of an outline framework for the 50+ Workbook;
5. discussion with the partners and selected target groups about the applicability of the key sections of the Workbook and to identify other relevant areas;
6. drafting a set of materials developed to explore these key areas;
7. critiquing of draft materials by partners, and
   - testing with key informants working in the field;
   - testing with 50+ individuals;
   - taking feedback on drafts.
8. producing a final draft that was translated and contextualized by the partners;
9. piloting materials in the five partner countries:
   - the piloting involved reviewing the utility of the materials with people aged 50+ from different sectors and with professional status;
   - feedback was taken on final draft and amendments made;
10. production of a final copy translated and contextualized into partner languages, and printed;
11. the creation of a web version of the Workbook.

This process was useful in ensuring transferability of the specifically designed activities across transnational borders. The process described above and implemented in this project to produce the 50+ Workbook and online resources seemed to be effective for the different European partners and their older workers, as judged by the evaluative feedback from their pilot groups.

Improving the development process for transnational resources

The developmental process used in the 50+ Europe project ensured the materials met the needs and issues of the sample 50+ populations and the advisers' perceptions of 50+ needs. It produced activities which were tested for their utility in enabling the target audiences in partner countries to manage changes associated with employment.

The results from the pilots indicated the materials were of help in enabling people to engage with their work options. Could this detailed and complex procedure for developing effective materials for 50+ older workers be improved? Possibly, we concluded, through an even more grounded and action research-based development process. This could build on the activities collaboratively with people who are aged 50+. Obviously, since people have different learning styles, cultures and preferences for learning a wide range of activities would be needed. This approach could lead to a toolkit of materials, where selection would be made according to the specific needs and preferences of the group or individual.

It is possible that this action research format and grounded process would lead to a more thoroughly applicable educational resource with wider transferability. Such a resource could work most effectively with a generic core of broader international and educational transferability and subsidiary units or modules, to have specific applicability for a national partner to use with designated groups, or in specific situations.

This idea would need further piloting and it could ensure greater applicability and relevance to a wide range of transnational target audiences, assuming the original target groups were representative of this range. This action research and grounded process of development would add an individualized element, which would embrace local diversity, while also creating a generic core with wide applicability across diverse countries and groups. Whether this development process would be more time-consuming or difficult will partly depend on the need for localization within a partner country. For the process to work effectively, there may need to be a segmentation of the market, or a focusing on the specific groups that would benefit most from the initiative. This arguably should be happening anyway. Then the local participative and collaborative (target) groups could be established, designed to embrace the inherent diversity, with people from the target populations. This development model is based on initiatives from action research community development.

The materials produced in the 50+ Europe project

The 50+ Workbook materials were designed to support those over the age of 50 to identify their needs and priorities, build confidence and self-esteem, and suggest ways forward. They take into account different types of employment situation, including use with three different audiences:

1. job seeker – those seeking new employment;
2. job changers – those wishing to change their job;
3. job retainers – those who wish to remain with the same employer, and may want a different structure or role.

For each of the three audiences, core and optional materials were available. The materials for job changers are illustrative of the process. They included, for example, the observation that a starting point for any audience is to enable them to identify their needs and priorities. The key questions asked for this purpose included: What is important to you? What gives you fulfilment? What roles do you have? What needs do you have? These are fundamental questions in any life change management process, and extend the excellent work of Covey et al. (1999). The answers to these questions act as a foundation on which each person can build the next steps of their life.

After identifying priorities, a person would go on to identify their current needs, and then their feelings about their situation. This provides the agenda and the emotional context into which the needs fit. The materials were designed to move from generic to the specific needs so people then proceed to consider the practical activities involved in reviewing their work options.

The next themes to be developed relate to the specific qualities brought by the individual such as their strengths, qualities, skills and competences, qualifications and experience. These are then applied to the individual's prospective job interests and requirements.

The next step seeks to identify job requirements. This includes type of work, place of work, income, promotion prospects and levels of responsibility required. Once individuals have confirmed these important priorities, they are then in a position to focus on the more basic aspects of job change such as the job application process, preparing for interview and action planning. In this way the user of the material is able to build practical ways forward.

Potential difficulties or barriers encountered by 50+ job-seekers, such as maintaining motivation under failure to get paid work, are dealt with by building the potential solutions into core activities within the materials. It was during piloting with unemployed older workers, and with agencies supporting individuals in job-seeking, that many of these aspects had been identified and included. It was a key purpose of the pilot work to identify the barriers encountered by 50+-year-olds, and to seek to identify practical and realistic ways to overcome these.

Intergenerational Portfolio Management

The second EU project funded through the Leonardo da Vinci programme considered in this chapter was the Intergenerational Portfolio Management (IPM) (2006–2008). This project was designed to explore issues common to older and younger workers and specifically to extend the working lives of nurses and health care assistants (HCAs). This is a transnationally recognized need and area of labour shortage (see Chapter 11). This project focused on developing understandings of older nurses and HCAs about their working lives.

A key part of the process was bringing together older and younger nurses and HCAs to work in a co-mentoring way to identify:

- existing education, knowledge, skills and competencies for work;
- interests, skills and competencies developed outside the workplace;
- job satisfaction and frustrations;
- self-reflection on the meaning of their life and work planning for the nurses and HCAs;
- further training needs.

The IPM project was developed in Austria, Czechoslovakia, Greece, the Netherlands and the UK, and elaborated on curriculum vitae (CV)/personal portfolio-building. It also identified key training needs, which may be helpful in ensuring job satisfaction and helping to secure later life working. The IPM projects complemented the 50+ Europe project and supported many EU governments' intentions to extend working life.

Evaluation and feedback from the nurses and HCAs on the pilot project identified beneficial aspects for their co-mentoring activities. Some effects of the IPM project were immediate. The nurses/HCAs in their paired mentoring got to know each other better; they understood more about each other's work roles, ways of working, experiences and difficulties. They sought to resolve work problems and dilemmas together. This had the effect of improving working relationships and teamworking. If this was extended throughout a hospital, the researchers argued that it would positively influence the quality of patient care, job satisfaction, performance, and the targets reached by the health service.

Early evidence from the UK pilot showed that some nurses/HCAs had benefited from the process (Chiva et al. 2007). They reported feeling more valued, understood their colleagues and work environment better, could see themselves staying in their health service jobs longer, and recognized the value of building their electronic portfolios as a professional process. In the UK, professional portfolios are required for registration by the Nursing and Midwifery Council (NMC).

Some specific benefits identified by the nurses included:

- In terms of the nurse partnerships: exchange of Information between nurses/HCAs with different training backgrounds; and an opportunity to work with someone not normally part of the same team.
- In terms of personal professional needs: recognize own skills/ weaknesses; recognize training needs; identified the positive aspects of a previously interpreted negative trait; and 'opened eyes' to training needs.

- In terms of portfolios: updating personal portfolios; useful as a draft to develop and update the portfolios; and contribute future NMC portfolio/online.

For the project to be successful, some key elements were identified as important. In terms of nurse structures and hierarchies, these were a high awareness of the IPM process by managers; and careful selection and invitation of nurses/HCAs to work together. In terms of an allocation of time for nurse partners to work together with management support, people acknowledged the problems of a lack of time, and that specific time needed to be allocated and protected within the nurse duties to ensure that nurses/HCAs could attend each workshop. An easily accessible website was called for and one that should be available from the beginning of the project. This could helpfully contain a step-by-step guide to using the website and how to create e-portfolios. It should be easy to update and should contain text boxes without word limits.

The nurses/HCAs identified potential benefits for the hospital teams and hospital as a whole which included improved teamwork and the opportunities to identify training needs.

In terms of the hospital as a whole, they suggested that IPM portfolio development could be combined with other human resource and appraisal processes, and that this would improve and raise the profile of the NHS Trust internationally.

The IPM process was identified by the nurses/HCAs, their managers and local coordinators as having applicability across professional groups working in health services and across different diversity strands apart from age. The IPM process was considered to be a complementary process to existing HR and appraisal systems. It could provide the opportunity for HR and training managers to electronically draw together staff training needs.

Integrating Work and Retirement 'a call to action' – ways of managing later life Transitions, work and money

The Department of Work and Pensions (DWP) in the UK, recognizing the financial imperatives of underfunded retirement, established some pilot projects to influence savings by people in later life. It funded a small study (September 2006–March 2008) involving eight workshops held for employees from a range of work sectors, including midwives and other health service professionals, national and local charities, two housing associations in Wales, to enable people to review their work, retirement plans and money options. The content of the workshops included:

- Needs and issues concerning retirement and money including concerns and issues of the workshop participants; the changing retirement and pension landscape; and what to avoid as a pensioner.
- Reviewing the transition including visions and dreams; managing change model; work, relationships and leisure time working longer–maintaining skills and effectiveness.
- Financial capability including attitudes to money and money at different life stages; managing money–budgeting and debt; state pensions and benefits; occupational and personal pensions; pension changes in April 2007; taxation; savings and investment; risk and the risk pyramid; and obtaining advice.
- Focus on Health and Wellbeing
    - Additional support including: What do you need? Where from? By whom? And Signposting.
    - Motivation and life planning: taking action including identifying personal gaps and priorities, and organizing them for action.

The rationale was that these issues were important to enable older workers to manage their life changes effectively. This rests on an approach which has been well tested and has produced significant impacts (Royston 2007), the managing change model developed by Allin Coleman (Coleman and Chiva 1992). The model is a problem-solving strategy which can be applied generically to any change (see Figure 9.1).

The model in addition to being rational-logical, like other problem-solving models, incorporates an emotional intelligent element. The model during these workshops was modified to take into account two conceptual shifts: the need to plan earlier in life; and the trend to use the term 'life planning', rather than pre-retirement or retirement planning. Earlier retirement planning may not involve the anticipation of an abrupt change (see Figure 9.1).

The model has been successfully used for older workers, people in midlife and for those facing changes at other ages (Life Academy 2007). To use the model generically, a number of questions needed to be added to each step (see Figure 9.2).

Step one – the model can then be applied to any period of life, to changes or transitions, to needs, issues, problems and concerns and will enable people to manage more successfully. For any theme identified by the older worker, each step can be applied, whether to maintain employability or find work; flexibly retire or phase retirement; maintain health; review finances, time, or life purpose; or enhance relationships.

Step two – *taking stock* – specifically includes emotional intelligence. To complement the managing change model, Allin Coleman introduced a

Figure 9.1 Life planning model

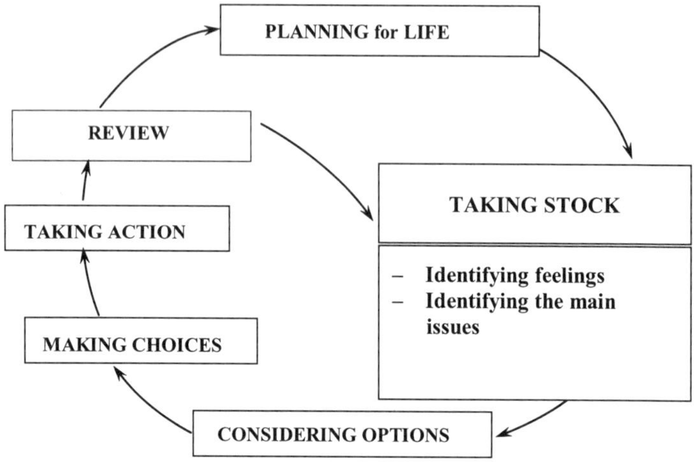

Source: Adapted from Coleman and Chiva (1992).

Figure 9.2 Applying the life planning model

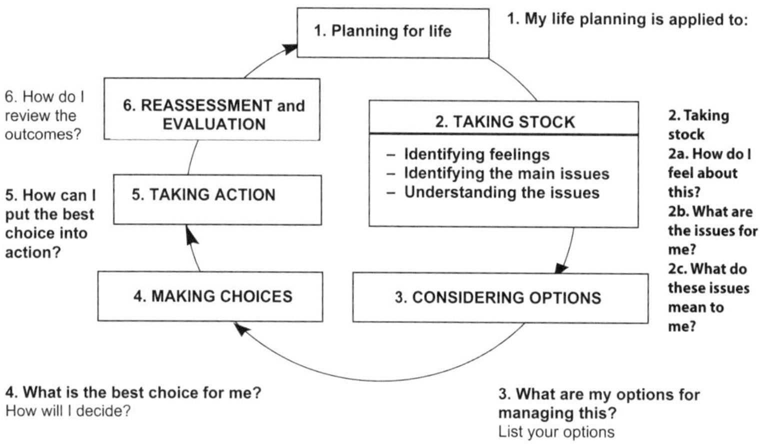

'feelings curve' (based on the work of Leone Sugerman and Elizabeth Kubler-Ross) (see Figure 9.3). Changes and losses (whether perceived or not) cause a sequence of thoughts and feelings. Any change, large or small, evokes these thoughts and feelings. This is a natural process and people have experienced these feelings many times in their lives. Typically, the pattern of thoughts and feelings experienced during changes are shock or euphoria, searching, anger, guilt, self-doubt, gradual acceptance and transition completed. Patterns of thoughts and feelings may vary slightly from change to change, or person to person. For example, a person may 'miss out' one or two of the stages in the transition.

Another common effect is to 'stall' in one part of the curve, going over the same thoughts or feelings again and again (see Figure 9.3). Eventually, after a period of time, which can vary from seconds to several years, the change will be completed.

Figure 9.3 Feelings curve

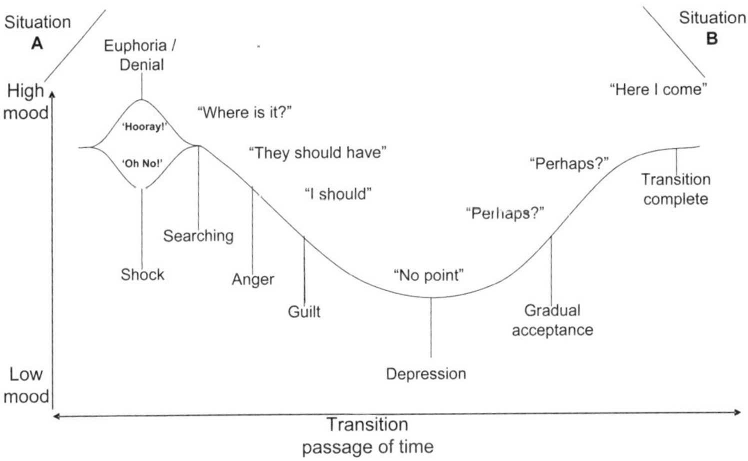

A detailed evaluation process was used for the Integrating Work and Retirement Workshops in the Call to Action Programme (including pre-course, post-course and three-month post-course follow-up questionnaires). This demonstrated that significant actions had been taken by the participants up to three months after the workshop when they completed their final evaluation (Royston 2007):

- 59% of respondents had obtained a forecast of their state pension;
- 77% had looked at their occupational/personal pension fund statement and forecast;
- 45% had sought financial planning advice;
- 45% had increased their savings/investments for retirement;
- 25% of those eligible had increased their contributions to their pension;

- 27% had changed their intentions about retirement (with the majority intending to work longer).

Clearly, the interim results from this project suggest the effectiveness of the workshops in many areas of people's lives, including reviewing savings, pensions, retirement plans and health.

Summary

The three projects, 50+ Europe, Intergenerational Portfolio Management and Integrating Work and Retirement, were all based on ways of engaging older workers and their employers to harness older people's potential. The models and approaches used in these projects built on work developed in change management and life planning preparation over three decades.

The processes built on individual competence, the ability and desire to manage change and empower the individual in their work-life choices. In terms of educational methodologies, these three projects included self-facilitated (self/individual), peer-facilitated and group-facilitated learning. These forms of learning all played their part in developing deeper understandings of later-life working; the contribution of reflections on career, work, and managing transitions into any life change, such as retirement.

Bibliography

Beck, U. (1998) Politics of risk society, in J. Franklin (eds) *The Politics of Risk Society*. Cambridge: Polity Press.

Biggs, S. (1999) *The Mature Imagination: Dynamics of Identity in Midlife and Beyond*. Milton Keynes: Open University Press.

Bridges, W. (1995) *Managing Transitions*. London: Nicholas Brealey Publishing.

Centre for Research on the Older Worker (CROW) (2004) *Changing Work in Later Life: A Study of Job Transitions*. Guildford: University of Surrey.

Centre for Senior Planning (2004) *Norway Senior Barometer*. Oslo: Centre for Senior Planning.

Centre for Senior Planning (2005a) Program for the *International Research Conference. Promoting Active Ageing in Work Life*, Oslo 2–3 June.

Centre for Senior Planning (2005b) *Audit Tool*. Oslo: Centre for Senior Planning.

Centre for Senior Planning (2005c) *The Senior Planning Audit.* Oslo: Centre for Senior Planning.

Chiva, A., Shepherd, J. and Humphreys, C. (2003) A theoretical perspective on vocational guidance. Paper presented at the *Ageing Societies: Critical Perspectives on the Past, Present and Future, British Society of Gerontology* 34th Annual Scientific Meeting, Keele University, 14–16th July 2005.

Chiva, A., Shepherd, J. and Howard, M.F. (2007) Workshop paper: benefits of age Intergenerational Portfolio Management to *Equality and Diversity Conference November 2007.* London: NHS Employers.

Coleman, A. and Chiva, A. (1991) *Coping with Change: Focus on Retirement.* London: Health Education Authority.

Coleman, A. and Chiva, A. (1992) *Managing Change: Focus on Retirement.* London: Health Education Authority.

Covey, S.R., Merrill, A.R. and Merrill, R.R. (1999) *First Things First.* New York: Simon & Schuster, Inc.

Department of Work and Pensions (DWP) (2002) *Simplicity, Security and Choice: Working and Saving for Retirement.* London: The Stationery Office.

Department of Work and Pensions (DWP) (2005) *Opportunity Age.* London: The Stationery Office.

Department of Work and Pensions (DWP) (2006) *Personal Accounts: A New Way to Save.* London: The Stationery Office.

European Union (UN) (2006) *Directive 2000/78/EC Prohibiting Discrimination in Employment.* Brussels: EU.

Hagan Hennessy, C. and Walker, A. (2004) *Growing Older: Quality of Life in Old Age.* Maidenhead: McGraw-Hill.

Hirsch, D. (2003) *Crossroads After 50.* York: Joseph Rowntree Foundation.

Jung, C. (1967) *Collected Works.* London: Routledge and Kegan Paul.

Life Academy (2007) *Applying the Life Planning Model to Themes of Change,* Professional Training Workshop, 23 January, Guildford.

McNair, S. and Flynn, M. (2005) *The Age Dimension of Employment Practice: Employer Case Studies* 42. London: Department of Trade and Industry.

Phillipson, C.R. (1998) *Reconstructing Old Age: New Agendas in Social Theory and Practice.* London: Sage Publications.

Phillipson, C.R. (2002) *Transitions from Work to Retirement: Developing a New Social Contract.* Bristol: The Policy Press.

Philipson, C. (2004) Work and retirement transitions: changing sociological and social policy contexts, *Social Policy and Society*, 3(2): 155–62.

Rogers, C. (1961) *On Becoming a Person*. Boston: Houghton Hofflin.

Rogers, C.R. (1986) A Client-centered/Person-centered Approach to Therapy, in I. L. Kutash and A. Wolf (ed.) *Psychotherapist's Casebook: Theory and Technique in the Practice of Modern Times*. San Francisco: Jossey-Bass.

Royston, S. (2007) Can education influence and motivate individuals to action? *Journal for the Professional Management Institute*, June: 14–15.

Taylor, P. (2002) ***New Policies for Older Workers***. Bristol: Policy Press.

Taylor, P. (2006) *Employment Initiatives for an Ageing Workforce in the EU-15*. Luxembourg: Office for Official Publications of the European Communities.

Vincent, J. A., Phillipson, C.R. and Downs, M. (2006) *The Futures of Old Age*. London: Sage Publications.

Walker, A. (2005) (ed.) *Growing Older in Europe*. Maidenhead: Open University Press/McGraw-Hill.

Worsley, R. and Moynagh, M. (2002) *The Opportunity of Lifetime: Reshaping Retirement*. King's Lynn: The Tomorrow Project.

10 Making the most of experience – the East Midlands story

Elizabeth Farmer and Jim Soulsby

National recognition of the issues and challenges of the ageing UK (United Kingdom) working population and local recognition of the potential impact on the skills and economy of the East Midlands region of England resulted in the funding of the Mature Workforce Initiative by the East Midlands Regional Development Agency in 2000. This initiative brought together a number of organizations that had been raising awareness of the developing skills and demographic challenge for employers; projects that had developed positive and practical solutions for people aged over 45 who wanted to work; and processes for recognizing and valuing the experience and skills of older workers and learners. This unique local, regional and national partnership that became Experience Works! in 2002 developed a brand that spoke both to people aged over 45 and employers, and came to the attention of policy-makers in the UK and the rest of Europe.

As the working population in the UK grows older, older people often face the challenges of early exit from the workplace and threats to the security of their pensions (Department for Work and Pensions (DWP) 2002a). Their efforts to find work, or change career, have often faltered for lack of confidence and failure to recognize, value and market their skills and experiences effectively (Centre for Research into the Older Worker (CROW) 2004). Long before English age discrimination legislation in 2006, many older job-seekers felt their age was against them and that age discrimination, real or imagined, was rife. Indeed, many employers had used age as a determinant for redundancy and the cultures of early retirement dominated not only the public sector but also traditional manufacturing and old engineering sectors that struggled for survival through the 1980s and 1990s (see Chapter 2).

Public policy spoke of the need to employ older workers and increasingly for people to work longer, to fund the social costs of longer life expectancy and higher expectations of retirement. Employers battled with skills shortages, unfilled vacancies and inexperienced management, while older people retired at or before pension age taking large chunks of corporate memory with them and the mistaken belief they were making way for the younger generation persisted (DWP 2006; CROW 2004).

There appeared to be a gap between expectation and practice and a gap in the services targeted at the mature worker and job-seeker. Experience Works! grew out of a desire to develop and customize a best practice approach to empower mature people to stay in work longer and to find for themselves new work in a radically changed labour market, to have their experience recognized and to get that work by their own merits. This was not only because employers were under pressure to employ older workers but because older people could demonstrate the value they brought.

It was not only what Experience Works! did but how it did it that was innovative. This included the active participation of older people in the design, development and evaluation of the process together with the active engagement of local, regional, national and European partners, policy-makers and supporters at every stage (Experience Works 2001a).

Why we did it

Work with and for older workers started in Loughborough College in the mid-1990s when it was realized that older people who were being made redundant faced difficulty in re-entering the labour market because of their lack of familiarity with that labour market, lack of confidence in their abilities, an inability to recognize and value their experience, and their lack of skills in marketing themselves to new employers (Ford and Soulsby 2001). In the relatively low-skill East Midlands region, this particular group of workers from old manufacturing and engineering industries, post-war baby boomers who were turning 45 in the early 1990s had started work in the 1960s and 1970s, and expected to work until retirement like their parents. In many cases they expected to remain with the same employer. They had first entered the employment market when there was a choice of jobs; they could leave one job on a Friday and walk into another one on a Monday. Often working in the same organization as their fathers, they had never been through any recruitment and selection processes. It was not unusual for people aged over 45 to have never written a curriculum vitae (CV) or to have had a job interview. Not only were they facing the trauma of redundancy, they also faced the challenge of finding another job in a rapidly changing world of work. With the decline of traditional industries, the development of new technology and globalization, older people found their qualifications were unrecognized, their skills were out of date, current recruitment practices were unfamiliar, and existing agencies, the recruitment industry and some human resource professionals could not understand what the problem was and were insensitive to the failure of older people to compete effectively in the labour market.

Developing a local response

The European Social Fund, under the Human Resource Adapt strand, was targeted at the employability of people aged over 45 in the labour market in the mid-1990s. Loughborough College successfully bid for these funds and developed, first, a 10-week accredited process for people aged over 45 who wanted to return to work (1995–97) and, second, a peer mentor training programme (1997–2000) (Ford and Soulsby 2001). From 2000–2002, funding from the East Midlands Development Agency (EMDA) brought together a larger regional partnership, the Mature Workforce Initiative that drew together two partnerships, Experience Works! (Loughborough College and New College Nottingham) and Mature Connections (Nottingham Training and Enterprise Council (TEC) and the Third Age Employment Network). Additional funding from UK Online and the European Social Fund enabled the establishment of two Experience Works! centres (one at Loughborough College and the other at New College Nottingham) (Mature Workforce Initiative 2001). These centres offered a customized service to people aged over 45 who wanted to learn, find work and stay there in a professional work environment, supported by mature professionals and peer mentors. From 2002–2004, the Experience Works! (the new name for the regional partnership) was rolled out with the appointment of five county coordinators who were hosted by the Learning and Skills Councils in each of the East Midland counties and the establishment of Experience Works! venues and workshops in Derbyshire, Nottinghamshire, Northamptonshire and Lincolnshire.

Micro-processes and partnerships

The initial 10-week process developed between 1995 and 1997 included job search, confidence building, work placement, information communication technology skills and brought people aged over 45 together in small groups working with mature people who had training, human resource, recruitment, general management and outplacement experience. The 15-hours-a-week programme, accredited by the Open College Network, was tested with people from diverse educational, work and social backgrounds. The main result of the project was that people regained their self-respect and confidence. They gained an IT (information technology) qualification; they found work they wanted, and they found this work themselves. The workshop activities, the development of self-appraisal, presentation and interview skills, practical peer appraisal and team-building ethos of the programme provided support, networks and friends who were in the same position but who were not competitors.

This project worked closely with the government Job Centre but clearly filled a gap in its service. There was no waiting period, no compulsion and no conflict with the Job Centre requirement to be available for work. Many of the clients were not eligible for Job Centre services or had had negative experiences of them. The return to learning often encouraged them to seek other qualifications. The development of a portfolio of evidence had the advantage of demonstrating the progress of the self-awareness process, the personal communication and marketing progress of CVs and letters, as well as the reality and progress of the job search. There were two inherent dangers in this approach – first was the production of the portfolio becoming more important than the job search – bad for the individual but good for the college which benefited from retention and achievement funding – and second – the person concerned getting a job before the portfolio or qualification was completed – great for the individual but bad news for the college. This became the central dilemma – the tension between getting a job and getting a qualification in how to get a job!

The 45+ Strategy for Positive Change was a European-funded transnational ADAPT project from 1997–2000. Working with Adulta College in Finland, the University of Antwerp in Belgium, and under the banner of AGE (Achievement and Growth lead to Employability) the partners looked at different ways of recognizing and valuing experience and skills in people aged over 45. In Loughborough, a Peer Mentoring Training package was developed and tested. In Antwerp groups of mature trade union representatives without formal education were trained, and they also looked at methods of accreditation of prior learning and experience with partners. In Strasbourg, in particular, the value of a French system for modelling changes in career direction (the ROME) was explored. Meanwhile, in Finland, people who had retired early were encouraged to return to work and develop new skills.

The Loughborough Peer Mentoring Training pack was developed with, by and for people aged over 45, who had experienced career change, midlife job search and were dedicated to the concept of lifelong learning. It was tested in the UK with a number of older job-seekers in college and older learners in company locations and delivered to individuals and groups. It was also tested on a European audience of trainers and employees of the Ministry of Employment as well as with trade union officers in Brussels. Local partners included the University of the Third Age, the Leicestershire branch of the then Institute of Personnel and Development; the Leicester-based

Employment National Training Organisation and the then Leicestershire TEC. A small but dedicated steering group had the advantage of looking local but being national. The members of this group were senior in their organizations, could make decisions, but, more importantly, took part in the development of the materials and the training, the review and evaluation as well as the visits to Finland and Brussels. They also actively engaged the other members of their organization in the participation, evaluation and promotion not only of the project but also of the business case for the engagement of older workers and the influencing of government policy. The final dissemination of the AGE project in Brussels in December 2000 attracted the interest of the UK Department of Work and Pensions and its Age Positive Team in Sheffield.

The main conclusion of the *45+ A Strategy for Positive Change* report (Ford and Soulsby 2001) was that positive action by people aged over 45 and a customized support service had a huge motivational effect on individuals and empowered them to learn, gain new skills and get the work they wanted for themselves. To date all the work with older people in colleges had taken place in a busy further education college geared very much to the 16–19 age groups. This often meant being subject to constant room changes and movement about the college surrounded by young people often aged 14–19 and generally aged about 16. This did not allow the customer-focused advantages of the process to be maintained and in some cases the age range was intimidating both for older and younger 'learners'.

The next premise was to test if a mature environment in a purpose-designed centre, staffed by and for mature job-seekers and learners, made a difference, and if that difference was also that of a workplace as opposed to a college environment. Loughborough College and New College Nottingham worked together to bid for funding from the East Midlands Development Agency, Skills Development Fund, to establish an Experience Works! centre at both colleges and to test out the above hypotheses in both city centre and market town locations.

While Loughborough College had been developing a service for mature job-seekers and learners, the Third Age Employment Network (TAEN) – now The Age and Employment Network, established in 1997, had been active in the East Midlands raising awareness of the challenges faced by older workers (for more on TAEN, see Chapter 7). In particular, it had been working in Nottingham to set up 'Mature Connections', a telephone helpline for people aged over 50, linking them to learning and work opportunities offered by partners across the city. A regional conference in 1999 with the title 'Age Works' launched a TAEN East Midlands Forum with members from across the region. By 2000, Nottingham TEC and TAEN were also seeking funding to extend and develop Mature Connections.

At this point, senior officers in the Regional Development Agency were excited at the possibility of developing the skills of local older workers. They saw the potential for the region of encouraging mature workers to stay in work longer at the same time as policy-makers began to realize the significance of the relative shortage of younger people entering the workforce, and the impact of the retirement of huge numbers of baby boomers from 2006 onwards. At the instigation of the Regional Development Agency, the Experience Works! and Mature Connections teams were invited to work together to produce a regional Mature Workforce Initiative.

This decision signalled an intention by the Regional Development Agency to take the skills of the ageing workforce seriously and a desire to develop a strategic regional approach. It gave the two partnerships a chance to work and think together and to develop a joint vision, with joint aims and objectives, as well as to budget and undertake some initial planning. The decision came at the same time as news of the successful funding bids by New College Nottingham and Loughborough College from UK Online and the European Social Fund that gave the colleges the challenge and the opportunity of equipping the Experience Works! centres with the latest technology and supporting people who came to the centres but who did not generate income for the colleges if they did not take qualifications.

The Mature Workforce Initiative (2001), managed by Elizabeth Farmer at Loughborough College, brought together a large regional network; two colleges with experience of the widening participation agenda, and two very positive and practical approaches to the dilemmas faced by older learners, workers and job-seekers – the successful model developed by the Loughborough team for 45+, and the telephone helpline for people aged over 50 in Nottingham. The new regional steering group represented these different strands and also brought together key regional players, expert agencies and national organizations. Members included the DWP, the Confederation of British Industry (CBI), the Trades Union Congress (TUC), Government Office East Midlands (GOEM), the Learning and Skills Council (LSC), Job Centre Plus (JCP), the East Midlands Regional Local Government Association (EM-RLGA), Learn Direct, Better Government for Older People (BGOP), TAEN, NIACE as well as the Development Agency and the two colleges. This provided the Development Agency with the unexpected bonus of supporting the first regional initiative in the UK on the ageing workforce, based on well-researched work and established networks linking into the national political agenda. Furthermore, the involvement of so many national and regional partners, the commitment of the members and the level at which they operated and influenced policy, raised the Experience Works! profile and expectations at a time when the issue of older workers was reaching the public policy agenda.

From 2000–2002, the key objectives were to develop the two centres in Loughborough and Nottingham for people aged over 45 with customized support to return to or stay in work, to develop the Mature Connections helpline in Nottingham and to raise awareness across the East Midlands of the issues and challenges of the ageing workforce. Several factors combined to turn the spotlight on the East Midlands's efforts – policy concern at the number of people aged over 50 reliant on Incapacity Benefit and Job Seekers Allowance, government determination to get them back to work, the emergence of the extending working life agenda as the pensions crisis deepened, and the hint of age discrimination legislation (DWP 2006; TAEN 2006).

The Mature Workforce Initiative's development of practical solutions and the success of attracting people aged over 45 to the centres and those aged over 50 to the telephone helpline demonstrated a need for advice and information. They also highlighted that government agencies were not reaching certain older workers and that many older job-seekers and career changers were not finding the services they needed, despite a plethora of agencies offering services and support which it was assumed mature people wanted or needed (TAEN 2007).

The Experience Works! centres were developed to be working environments, with brand new technology, experienced tutors, mentors and customer-designed and evaluated programme that valued and recognized the experiences of older people, whatever their background. The centres were a repository for practical solutions to their fears and perceived shortcomings and they provided positive strategies for the regaining of confidence, the development of new skills, and the assured move into work that they were happy with, further qualifications or continued learning.

The other main feature of Experience Works! was flexibility. People could join a structured 10-week programme, have one-to-one consultations, attend without appointment and undertake many activities or just a few, or just work in the centre, making use of its seminar rooms, small consultation rooms, open-plan computer suites, with opportunities for individual or small group learning, wireless technology, white boards, flat screens, and so on. These recognized that older people should have the best equipment and not the oldest and the worst as so often used to happen for a generation that had started work when computers took huge space in specially air-conditioned suites, and when they were seen as a specialist function and were not omnipresent at work and home. The older generation often were unfamiliar with technical IT programmes and had engaged slowly and often reluctantly with them. Many, consequently, were looking for work later in their lives without the experience or confidence of working with IT and this, in itself, was often used by employers as examples of the inflexibility of older workers, their reluctance to learn and their resistance to change.

Both centres had separate entrances on the main college sites and were staffed with people who had experienced redundancy and major career change and who had worked across sectors, at different levels, had different educational attainments and qualifications, had moved in their careers and were altogether credible role models. This enabled the centres to cater for people from all sorts of background; people who had been out of work for some time, returners, people with no skills, low skills, managers and senior managers, and people who had worked for themselves. Among the tutors, mentors, centre staff and peers there was always someone who understood people's backgrounds, knew the industry sector or organization they had worked in, could speak the same language and understood their hopes and fears.

The wide experience of the staff was reflected in the diversity of the client group. The power of the peer group cannot be underestimated. It replaced the social network and support lost from work, just as the centre replaced the workplace, and the training and job search replaced the work. More than that, working together in groups and through the Experience Works! process helped people identify what they were good at, what work they were looking for, where they wanted to work and gave them other pairs of eyes, helping hands, extended networks and contacts in other locations, most importantly without competing with each other because they were all looking for different sorts of work. Moreover, the peer group supported and encouraged the more timid, the shyer and less able, the less confident, the less skilled and those who had had fewer opportunities. Conversely, the groups also effectively dealt with antisocial, disruptive, arrogant or negative attitudes, so often displayed by disgruntled and aggrieved older job-seekers, more effectively than staff and mentors which resulted in shared responsibility for the success of the group and individual experience as well as a sense of caring, sharing and pulling together.

The name and the brand Experience Works! had the advantage of appearing independent, sending positive messages about the potential of the older workforce, reflecting the desire of people to choose how long they worked and the sort of work they did, and flagging up an issue and solution to employers facing not only a shortage of recruits but, more significantly, a shortage of people with the right skills and application. Both centres received many requests from employers for 'good older workers' and often people who successfully found work were asked to see if Experience Works! had more like them. Gradually employers began to use Experience Works! and to post vacancies at the centres, as well as using the service as part of their outplacement provision for redundancies.

Meanwhile, the Mature Connections coordinator, hosted by Nottingham City Council, developed a good practice guide for employers, worked with recruitment agencies and built on the city-wide partnership and referral network to support hundreds of people aged over 50 who were calling the helpline, and all had a story to tell about their alienation from the labour market, age discrimination and the challenges of finding work, support and targeted training and advice. A half-day conference in Nottingham in 2001 attracted 500 people aged over 50 who wanted an opportunity for their voices to be heard.

This phase of the mature workforce initiative was characterized by enthusiastic support from the Regional Development Agency, strong leadership from the chairperson, dedicated and participative steering group members and excellent partnership work with national partners. The success of the Experience Works! centres attracted the attention of the government Cabinet Office, especially in terms of older women, the DWP in relation to New Deal 50+ employment programme, and the Secretary of State for Pensions as part of the older people's agenda being developed by Better Government for Older People. The TAEN grew in numbers and influence and there was a strong desire from other East Midlands counties to share in the success of the Nottingham and Loughborough experiences.

The years 2002 to 2004 saw the regional rollout of Experience Works! (the Initiative was renamed to avoid confusion and to give a stronger image and impact). The national impetus in public policy, the work in the counties with the Third Age Employment Network and its growing network of partners led to each of the East Midlands counties hosting an Experience Works! coordinator to work with local organizations to develop Experience Works! centres and activity to meet the needs of older people and employers. In 2002 five county coordinators were appointed and local recruitment campaigns were launched in each county. These were people experienced in recruitment, training, public and private sector organizations, fund-raising with local knowledge, experience of career change and both enthusiasts and role models for the mature workforce (East Midlands Development Agency 2005).

The appointment of the county coordinators brought the possibility of Experience Works! centres and workshops to people who previously had not been able to travel to Loughborough and Nottingham. The regional team were determined to make the service available not only in the further education sector but other venues, in areas of particular deprivation, in community and business centres. Many tasters and workshops were held in different locations and with regional and local partners, and negotiations were held with many organizations that wished to offer an Experience Works! service. The addition to the team of a business development manager enabled the testing of different models of partnership, the training and development of new centre staff, the protection and development of the Experience Works! brand and image, and the development of a business plan looking at the feasibility of the sustainability of Experience Works! At the same time the website was further developed to enable online registration and referral, negotiations with Learn Direct looked at the potential of expanding the Nottingham helpline into a national service and interest in Experience Works! was being expressed in other regions.

Project decline

The expansion of the regional team, the enthusiastic uptake of Experience Works! in the counties and the expectation of the rollout of the Experience Works! service coincided with influences which meant that the successful public face of Experience Works! hid political, structural and funding tensions as people and organizations jockeyed to work with and against Experience Works! Key factors here were changes in the make-up, leadership and partnerships of the steering group, and the perceived reduced importance of the older workforce issue at the Regional Development Agency. Complex and growing initiatives or projects need political will, vision and courage, as well as a desire to share agendas and make partnerships work. Many of the original steering group members who had created the vision and tirelessly espoused the cause felt alienated and saddened by the reluctance of the further education sector, because of funding changes, to develop the vision and realize the potential of the project. Loughborough College still held the contract but felt unable to carry the risk of employing and managing a growing regional team any longer as its own funding changed radically with a shift in its focus to those mainly aged 14–19.

Ironically, as the Regional Development Agency strategy on the ageing workforce which had always been fragile became virtually invisible, the DWP was mapping RDA interest and engagement nationally and promoting Experience Works! as an example of good practice. Experience Works! had increasingly been managed as a separate project which was seen by many as having had more than its fair share of funding and success. The decision of Loughborough College to cease to be the contract holder in 2004 led not only to the disbanding of the regional team, the closure of the Experience Works! flagship centre at Loughborough College and eventually the centre at New College Nottingham, but also the loss of 10 years of experience in the successful empowerment of older learners and job-seekers. With the loss of strategic emphasis and vision, the closure of operational bases and the dissolution of networks came the end of the East Midland's perceived lead in the development of innovative and successful solutions to the challenges of the mature workforce.

Although the name lives on, it is now very difficult to find evidence of the ground-breaking approach that was Experience Works! Ironically, the very conditions which spurred the original partners to action are even more acute today. There are greater numbers of older people in the workforce, there are significantly fewer younger people entering the workforce, and many people who can afford to are leaving the workforce. The impact of age discrimination legislation on employers is still to be evaluated and older workers still feel discriminated against in the labour market. More significantly, many employers, especially smaller employers, have yet to recognize the future impact of the demographic changes and older people have yet to be convinced that that they will ever be recognized and valued in the labour market. At a time of rapid changes in employment practices, because of the availability of pan-European labour in England, the outstanding challenge of the role, fit and future of older workers in the East Midlands is still to be addressed.

Bibliography

Centre for Research into the Older Worker (CROW) (2004) *Changing Work in Later Life: A Study of Job Transitions.* Guildford: University of Surrey.

Christopolous, M. (2001) *Mature Connections Employers Directory, June 2001.* Nottingham: Mature Connections.

Department for Education and Employment (DfEE) (1999) *Age Diversity in Employment: A Code of Practice; Guidance and Case Studies.* London: Department for Education and Employment.

Department for Education and Science (DfES) (1998) *The Learning Age.* London: Department for Education and Science.

Department for Education and Science (DfES) (2003) *Challenging Age: Information, Advice and Guidance for Older Age Groups.* London: Department for Education and Science.

Department of Work and Pensions (DWP) (2001). *Putting Yourself in the Picture: New Deal 50 Plus Pamphlet.* London: Department of Work and Pensions.

Department of Work and Pensions (DWP) (2002a) *Older People: Statistical Information Booklet.* Sheffield: Department of Work and Pensions.

Department of Work and Pensions (DWP) (2002b) *Simplicity, Security and Choice: Working and Saving for Retirement.* London: The Stationery Office.

Department of Work and Pensions (DWP) (2006) *Personal Accounts: A New Way to Save.* London: The Stationery Office.

Development & Change (2001a) *The Mature Workforce Initiative: Second Research Report*, October. Nottingham: Development & Change, East Midlands Development Agency.

Development & Change (2001b) *Mature Workforce Initiative: Interim Evaluation of Mature Connections*, 11 June. Nottingham: Development & Change, East Midlands Development Agency.

Development & Change (DCS) (2001c) *Mature Workforce Initiative: Final Report and Evaluation*, December. Nottingham: Development & Change, East Midlands Development Agency.

East Midlands Development Agency (EMDA) (2001) *East Midlands Leads Britain in Defusing Demographic Time Bomb*, 12 January. Nottingham: East Midlands Development Agency Press Office.

East Midlands Development Agency (EMDA) Monitoring Systems (2005) *New Core Output and Additional KPI Definitions Version 1*, March. Nottingham: East Midlands Development Agency.

East Midlands Regional Development Association (2005) *East Midlands Regional Economic Strategy Consultation*, September. Nottingham: East Midlands Development Agency.

Employment Skills and Productivity Partnership (ESPP) (2006) *Summary of the Action Plan*. Nottingham: East Midlands Development Agency.

Experience Works! (2001–2002) *Newsletter Issues 2, 3, 4*. Loughborough: Experience Works!

Experience Works! (2001a) *Press Cuttings (1) – Quiet Storm*. Loughborough: Experience Works!

Experience Works! (2001b) *Press Cuttings (2)*. Loughborough: Experience Works!

Farmer, E. (2002) United Nations World Assembly on Ageing – 8–12 April, *Diary and Reflections*, Loughborough: Experience Works!

Ford, G. (1996) *Career Guidance for the Third Age: Invitational Policy Consultation*. A report of NICEC /CRAC. Cambridge: National Institute for Careers Education and Counselling.

Ford, G. (1997) *Career Guidance in the Third Age: A Mapping Exercise*. NICEC Project Report. Cambridge: National Institute for Careers Education and Counselling.

Ford, G. and Soulsby, J. (2001) *Mature Workforce Development – East Midlands 2000. Research & Report*, January. Leicester: NIACE.

Foresight Ageing Population Panel (2000) *The Age Shift: A Consultation Document*. London: Department of Trade and Industry.

Grattan, P., Ford, G., Soulsby, J. and Watkins, B. (2001) *Ageing to Advantage: Work, Learning and Guidance for Older Age Groups*. London: Third Age Employment Network.

Mature Workforce Development East Midlands (2000) *Research and Report: Summary of Key Findings and References*. Leicester: NIACE.

Third Age Employment Network (TAEN) (2001) *Ageing to Advantage: Work, Learning and Guidance for Older Age Groups*. London: Third Age Employment Network.

Third Age Employment Network (TAEN) (2006) *Facts and Figures on Pensions and Retirement*. London: Third Age Employment Network (www.taen.org.uk/resources).

Third Age Employment Network (TAEN) (2007) *Managing the Ageing Workforce: An Introductory Guide to Age Management for HR Professionals*. London: Third Age Employment Network (www.taen.org.uk).

11 The working experiences of older nurses and midwives in the NHS

Jo Aspland, Helen Gibson, Anne Stimpson, Roger Watson and Jane Wray

Introduction

The scarcity of qualified health personnel, including nurses and midwives, is being highlighted as one of the biggest obstacles to achieving the Millennium Development Goals (MDGs) of improving the health and well-being of the global population (Buchan and Calman 2004). In January 2004, the High Level Forum on the Health MDGs reported: 'There is a human resources crisis in health, which must be urgently addressed' (WHO 2004: 5). Buchan and Calman's 2006 study for the International Council of Nursing (ICN) looked at the global distribution of these nurses, employing a nurse to population ratio for various countries. Their findings show that Europe, as a developed and relatively rich region, has a nurse to population ratio 10 times that of Africa and South Asia. Within Europe, western Europe/Scandinavia has a ratio about twice that reported in the south-east of Europe; there are also marked variations within the western Europe/Scandinavia sub-region, with Scandinavian countries reporting nurse to population ratios much higher than Spain, Portugal and Greece (Buchan and Calman 2004).

Although, in global terms, Europe has a relatively high nurse to population ratio, it is, nonetheless, experiencing a nursing and midwifery shortage along with many other parts of the world. In a recent report on health systems, the Organization for Economic Co-operation and Development (OECD) highlighted that 'shortages have already appeared in a number of OECD countries' (OECD 2004: 12). HOPE, the European Hospital and Healthcare Federation, confirmed the occurrence of these shortages in many European countries (HOPE 2004).

One of the principal reasons identified for the shortage in industrialized nations is the ageing of the health care workforce. The labour market participation of older workers (i.e. those aged 50 years and over) continues to attract considerable attention, as the numbers in employment decline and those who are inactive or retired increase (Loretto et al. 2006). Against a background of concern over the economic and social implications of low employment rates among the over-50s, much public policy has come to focus on extending the average working life by encouraging people to work for longer and to delay retirement (e.g. House of Lords 2003).

The National Health Service (NHS) is the largest employer in the United Kingdom (UK). The largest group of employees within the organization is nurses and midwives, and this workforce is ageing. Between 1983 and 1998 the average age of working registered nurses increased by more than four years, from 37.4 years to 41.9 years (Buerhaus et al. 2000). In 1998, Buchan found that approximately one in five nurses in the UK was aged 50 or over, and by 2010 it is likely that this will change to one in four (Buchan 1998). In addition, intakes into the profession have reduced markedly in recent years and have a much broader age range than in previous decades.

Despite recruitment and retention initiatives, this sector of the workforce will experience a significant shortage, especially in primary care settings, as nurses and midwives retire (Buchan and Scccombe 2005). In March 2000, there were around 22,000 whole-time equivalent vacant posts in the NHS and of these 9,900 (or 45 per cent) had been vacant for three months or more (Buchan 2000). The size of the registered nursing workforce has been forecast to be nearly 20 per cent below projected requirements by 2020 (Buerhaus et al. 2000).

The age profile of nurses and midwives is variable across the sector, and the oldest age profile is of community staff nurses, health visitors and district nurses (Buchan and Seccombe 2005; Watson et al. 2003). There has been some growth within nursing, especially among nurse managers, first-level registered nurses and registered sick children's nurses, but health visiting and midwifery have encountered little growth and there is a reduction in growth for district nursing (Buchan and Seccombe 2005). The Royal College of Midwives (RCM) estimates that 10,000 more midwives are needed in the UK to deliver one-to-one care for new mothers. Many new midwives leave before being in practice for three years because of work pressures and staff shortages leaving fewer midwives to fill the gap left by retiring midwives (RCM 2006).

The significance of this ageing workforce is twofold. First, many nurses are reaching the middle or end of their careers and are likely to have different needs and attitudes to nursing work. Second, it is clear that greater numbers of nurses and midwives are reaching, or will soon be reaching, potential retirement age (Buchan 1999). The average age of a student nurse currently qualifying is 29 years compared with 20 or 21 years in the 1960s (Ball and

Pike 2005). The average age of students entering training to be midwives is 34, indicating a similar problem for midwifery (Royal College of Midwives (RCM) 2006). The work-life span of current nursing and midwifery recruits is, therefore, significantly shorter than in previous decades.

The shortage of nurses and midwives is likely to have a major impact on health care. Nursing shortages and understaffing have been linked to a range of negative outcomes including increased mortality rates; adverse events after surgery; increased incidence of violence against staff; increased accident rates and patient injuries; and increased cross infection rates (Buchan and Calman 2004). Between 1974 and 1989 there was a 22 per cent increase in acute in-patient admissions to hospitals (Victor and Khakoo 1994), and this continuing trend indicates that even more nurses and midwives will be needed to meet the greater demand for patient care.

Retention is a key issue for the British NHS in terms of cost. It costs about £34,000 to train a nurse (first-level entry) and £4,900 to recruit and induct a replacement (Newman et al. 2001). The Royal College of Nursing (RCN) estimates that because 30 per cent of trained nurses are out of the current workforce, an investment of £5 billion has already been lost (RCN 2001). In addition, the increasing cost of pensions is putting pressure on the NHS which has to bear much of the cost. The UK has seen a general increase in early retirement and it is now common for men and women to be leaving the workforce from 50 years old (Phillipson 1998). People are leaving the labour market with many active years in front of them and often seek alternative occupation, if not employment (Watson et al. 2003). A single transition from work to retirement at a standard age is no longer the norm.

Encouraging nurses to return to nursing is also important. Buchan (2000) estimated that there were over 70,000 registered nurses not employed in nursing in the UK. The majority of these nurses were aged 50 years or older, with only 7 per cent actively seeking employment in nursing. Between 1999 and 2002, an average of 3,700 nurses returned to practice each year (RCN 2003: 10). Given the current severe nursing shortage, the nursing profession could look at this source of nurses to address the problem (Hawley and Foley 2004).

In the NHS, many older nurses and midwives experience ill health in retirement, from illness and/or disability (Wray et al. 2006), often as a consequence of their work. It is estimated that the cohort of 5,469 NHS employees who retired early in 1998–9 will cost the Pensions Agency an additional £416 million up to the age of 70 than if they had retired at the usual age. The huge cost to the NHS could be reduced if redeployment were encouraged (Pattani et al. 2001), or if patient care delivery was made more ergonomically sensitive to an older workforce. Work-related injuries are a key concern for the NHS as they cost millions of pounds in terms of sickness absence each year (Pattani et al. 2001). The impact on the individual is equally substantial.

Research to date

In the last five years there has been substantial growth of research in the UK in the broad areas of the employment of older workers and retirement transitions (Loretto et al. 2006). The Joseph Rowntree Foundation's *Transitions After 50* programme sponsored a body of work which looked at many facets of the experience of older workers. These included income in later life (Bardasi and Jenkins 2002; Meadows 2002); employment transitions of older workers (Lissenburgh and Smeaton 2003; Watson et al. 2003); the organizational context of retirement (Vickerstaff et al. 2004); the impact of caring on work life (Mooney et al. 2002) and the lessons to be drawn from international experiences of age policies and discrimination legislation (Hornstein et al. 2001; Taylor 2002). The conclusions drawn from the programme as a whole were that older workers are a diverse group, facing multiple pressures, and often with limited control over the timing or manner of decisions about continuing or stopping work (Hirsch 2003, 2005). Despite the burgeoning literature on older workers, relatively little is known about the attitudes and expectations of those under scrutiny: older workers themselves (Loretto et al. 2006).

In one of the studies commissioned by the Joseph Rowntree Foundation under its *Transitions after 50* research programme, Watson et al. (2003) sought to explore the options, decisions and outcomes facing nurses aged over 50. The research team interviewed older nurses employed by the NHS, those outside the NHS, and those who had returned – or were considering returning – to the NHS; in addition, other stakeholders, including employers, advisers and policy-makers, were consulted. Watson and his colleagues identified factors affecting an older nurse's decision to stay in work, which included flexible hours, access to continuing professional development (CPD), personal caring commitments and financial status.

Meadows (2002) found that older staff leave the NHS because they feel they are under too much pressure and that increased workload, lack of recognition, a culture of long working hours, lack of staff and support, physical wear and tear, continual change and the critical way the media portray the NHS are contributing factors. Storey et al. (2007) suggested that retention might be improved if older nurses were to receive remuneration that better reflects experience and skills, and greater promotion opportunities within clinical nursing posts rather than having to move into management posts to increase their pay.

Watson et al. (2003) identified that the group of ageing nurses in their study experienced a range of discriminatory practice in the workplace. Discrimination took place by commission: negative attitudes were held based on stereotypical views of the ability of older nurses to adapt to new technologies and recent developments in the field and also on their physical ability to do the job. Discrimination also took place by omission: this was seen in relation to CPD policies and practice, return to practice initiatives and retirement and pensions advice. Despite employers and policy-makers recognizing the contribution that older nurses returning to the NHS could make to the current staffing crisis, there was little evidence of policy and practice reflecting this. A major requirement of nurses aged over 50 is personally relevant information about pensions, retirement, CPD and flexibility in their work; these findings are echoed by Storey et al. (2007).

Stakeholders in Watson et al.'s (2003) study identified reasons for older nurses leaving the workforce, including the pace of technological change and stress – the latter of these was mentioned by the older nurses themselves as a significant influence on the retirement decision. Some stakeholders admitted that they preferred employing younger nurses; however, generally employers voiced many positive views about older nurses in the workforce. Older nurses in the study did not feel they had experienced overt ageism from their employers; more often they felt pressure from colleagues to retire in order to open up a job for a younger person. Many of the older nurses interviewed felt they were coping well with the physical and mental demands of nursing over the age of 50.

Practice could be improved by implementing some or all of the following: acknowledging the valuable contribution older nurses and midwives make; addressing the needs of older nurses and midwives through CPD/return to practice initiatives; providing more information; making flexible working options more available without affecting pension provision; allowing older nurses and midwives to move to less stressful areas of practice; and for the NHS to work collaboratively with the independent sector (Watson et al. 2003).

Wray et al.'s study (2006), building on the work conducted by Watson et al. (2003), examined the experiences of older nurses and midwives in the NHS. The project, supported by the European Social Fund, employed a systematic literature review, a content analysis of NHS human resources policy documents, a questionnaire survey in NHS Trusts and Primary Care Trusts of nurses and midwives aged 50 and over (with a smaller subset of those under 50) and semi-structured telephone interviews involving some of the questionnaire respondents.

Despite the evidence of discrimination against older nurses and midwives found in the literature, Wray et al. (2006) found only one area that yielded significant results in relation to age and that was access to CPD.

Comparing older and younger nurses and midwives, they found that older nurses accessed fewer CPD activities and this result was statistically significant. Seventy-three per cent of the sample aged 50 and over had not accessed any CPD activities in the last two years compared with 27 per cent of the under-50 sample. These findings around age and CPD are replicated in other studies.

Buchan (1999) cited the lower participation rates of nurses aged 50 or over in CPD compared with younger cohorts. The extent to which this is due to a lack of commitment from nurses, lack of provision, or age discrimination on the part of employers is unknown, although some studies suggest that it reflects genuine discrimination against older workers (Watson et al. 2003; Meadows 2002). Green (1987) expressed the view that the multiple roles that many female nurses are required to fulfil to balance professional and personal commitments, play a major role in determining their level of involvement with CPD. However, it may well be that older nurses and midwives with their wealth of experience and knowledge choose to access fewer CDP activities or they do not feel that CDP activities offered are relevant to their needs (Wray et al. 2006).

Older nurses need viable and relevant career development opportunities if they are to be motivated to stay in work. Bjork et al. (2007) found that further education and one day or more scheduled for CPD positively related to Norwegian nurses' intent to stay in the workforce. The ageing of the nursing workforce, combined with the increasing emphasis on lifelong learning, represents a CPD 'double whammy' – more nurses will enter middle age and will be more and more years distant from the time of their initial education and training, qualifications and entry on the register (Buchan 1999). In recent years, older nurses have been the group least active in CPD; this has implications for the level, content and methods of delivery of CPD that in the future will have to take account of the different needs of older nurses and their different patterns of working.

Wray et al.'s (2006) interview data also revealed some interesting perspectives in relation to age. Of the older nurses and midwives interviewed, only two (out of 22) felt there were no advantages associated with being aged 50 years or over in the NHS. The majority felt that experience was a definite advantage of being an older nurse or midwife. As for the disadvantages of increasing age, respondents spoke of the greater physical toll of the work, of age-related health problems and of being more tired generally. Several respondents reported that as a result of increasing age they had become more cynical (or were perceived as being more cynical) in relation to change in the NHS.

Several respondents reported experiencing some form of discrimination or problem in the workplace; while some were directly related to age, most spoke of the perceived threat of age discrimination, rather than of direct experience of it. Although none of the respondents had experienced problems with regard to recruitment and selection, some felt that their age affected training, promotion and career development. The group that appear to be most disadvantaged were those who experienced ill health, particularly in relation to experiencing discrimination, barriers to accessing CPD, quality of life, and mental health and well-being.

Older nurses and midwives interviewed about their current working experience in the NHS reported substantial satisfaction in their work particularly in relation to working with clients/patients and with their colleagues. This finding is replicated by Storey et al. (2007), where nurses were found to value patient contact; this should be appreciated by managers and reflected in work opportunities. Nursing and midwifery were seen positively as worthwhile careers with clear opportunities (Wray et al. 2006). Conversely, workload, stress, paperwork and bureaucracy impacted negatively upon this experience (Wray et al. 2006) and reducing workload, administration and increasing resources are possible solutions to these difficulties (Sandall 1998).

A modern health service requires modern employment services (Department of Health 2000a). Ethnicity, disability and work-related illness seem to affect older nurses disproportionately, and legislation and guidance from the Department of Health, to some extent, reflects this. Initiatives such as *Improving Working Lives* are well intentioned but their effectiveness has yet to be identified (Storey et al. 2007); until managers and employers prioritize these initiatives, little will change. Many older nurses and midwives who have considerable expertise to offer the NHS may not wish to pursue the option of retirement if redeployment was an option, or the opportunity was available for part-time working without compromising pension benefits (Wray et al. 2006). The ability of managers to manage staff effectively (Meadows 2002) and to recognize the valuable contribution that older workers make can only improve retention. More management training for middle management could be one direction in which to pursue improvements in retention. As the NHS has recognized that poor staff management is a key to the turnover of staff, improving the quality of management needs to be identified as an issue. There is a strong business case to be made for NHS employers paying attention to the needs of their older employees.

An important challenge will be to respond to the differing attitudes and needs of older nurses and midwives in their 40s and 50s. They may have another potential 10 – 20 years of service to contribute. Great consideration may need to be given to the provision of appropriate working hours, career development opportunities and phased retirement benefits. Government policy relating to the NHS is promoting work practices and lifelong learning opportunities that are friendly to nurses and midwives. This will need to be underpinned by financial benefits; for example, greater flexibility within the NHS pension scheme. An examination of the way career ladders/pay structures can continue to reward older nurses and midwives who have reached the top of their increment scale would also be of benefit in retaining this valuable resource for the future (Buchan 1999).

Hirsch commented that the NHS seems to be on 'an apparent march ... towards an ever more severe staffing crisis, despite the available alternative of nurturing an already trained pool of older labour' (Hirsch 2003: 14). The continued employment of older nurses and midwives within the NHS is a testimony to their experience, commitment and resilience; qualities which appear to have been both underestimated and undervalued. They represent a valuable resource that is in danger of being lost from the NHS workforce. In the broad context of factors affecting the employability of older workers, legislation on age discrimination may only have minimal impact. What is more important is to foster a supportive, informative environment for older workers – Loretto et al. (2006) expressed the need for a holistic approach to consider the needs and wishes of older people in extending their working lives. It is vital that the voice of older people themselves remains at the forefront of the research and policy agenda.

The findings from Watson et al. (2003) and Wray et al. (2006) identify the importance of attending to the needs of older workers in the NHS – both as a partial solution to the staffing crisis, and for the rights and well-being of the older workers themselves.

Methodological problems

To date, little research has been carried out that specifically focuses on older nurses and midwives, although there is a key need for this type of research to address their specific needs. However, undertaking in-depth research with NHS employees is not without its difficulties. The Department of Health's Research Governance Framework for Health and Social Care aims to 'set out principles, requirements and standards; define mechanisms to achieve these; describe monitoring and assessment arrangements; and improve research and safeguard the public' (Department of Health 2005: 1).

Several researchers have reported on their experiences of conducting research in health and social care under the Research Governance Framework. Leese et al. (2005) reported on the progress of two studies conducted during 2003–4 and 2004–5. The first study comprised a national postal survey sent to all Primary Care Cancer Leads and all PCT Chief Executives in England; this was followed by telephone interviews with respondents in a sample of six PCTs (Leese et al. 2004). The second study concerned primary care nurses: postal questionnaires were sent to primary care nurses in four PCTs, followed by interviews with a sample of participating nurses. In both studies, patients were not participants. The Framework, set up to improve the quality of research and protect the public while minimizing bureaucratic processes (Salisbury et al. 2005), was actually found to be more bureaucratic than the previous ethical approval process (Leese et al. 2005).

The problems reported by Leese et al. (2005) included difficulties in identifying the Research Management of Governance (RM&G) organizations (especially in the first of the projects), and inconsistency in the RM&G application forms. A standard form has since been developed; however, its use is not mandatory. Other issues identified by Leese et al. as problematic relate to sponsors' letters, honorary contracts, references and health checks/ Criminal Record Bureau (CRB) checks on researchers. There was also some confusion over projects designated as 'audit'; audits do not require Research Governance approval, yet the line that separates audit from research is 'narrow and open to interpretation' (Leese et al. 2005: 496).

Leese et al. (2005) discussed the implications of the Research Governance process for the two research projects under study. With regard to time, the process for the first project took six months and 50 per cent of a researcher's time over this period. The second study, although smaller and expected to be less problematic, disappointingly took the same amount of time. Leese et al. suggested that, based on their experience, conducting a national survey would be a near impossible task and would require a full-time person for six months just to get Research Governance approval. The implications of this for staffing and funding costs are obvious.

Kielmann et al. (2007) reported their experience of working on a project using telephone interviews targeting health service managers in a sample of Primary Care Organizations. The team used the R&D application form (Form D), designed to streamline applications for multi-centre research (Kielmann et al. 2007: 234). The project schedule dictated that these interviews took place over a period of three months. However, an estimated 318 staff hours were spent achieving R&D approval, requiring all the project's secretarial time, a substantial proportion of the senior researcher's time, and considerable input from the principal investigator, over a period of 10 weeks. Kielmann et al. found obtaining approval for this very low risk, multi-centre descriptive study involving NHS staff a 'cumbersome and time-consuming' process (2007: 236). Despite meticulous planning, the process threw the project into delay, threatened staff morale and adversely impacted on time for analysis, reviewing literature and preparing for subsequent phases of the study (Kielmann et al. 2007). Continuing requests for progress reports delayed the project further.

Elwyn et al. (2005), in their tellingly entitled paper 'Ethics and research governance in a multi-centre study: add 150 days to your study protocol', reported on a multi-centre study they had conducted using patient questionnaires. Achieving approval in all 20 NHS trusts to which they applied took a total of 103 days. A key factor in the time taken for approval for such multi-centre studies is the devolution of research governance to individual trusts, with a lack of central guidance, leading to diverse local interpretations and procedures (Kielmann et al. 2007).

Leese et al. (2005) also felt that the inclusion of NHS staff in the requirements to be unnecessary; this stipulation reduces the quality of research that can be reasonably undertaken. The second study by Leese et al. involved sending postal questionnaires to all practice nurses, district nurses, school nurses and health visitors in six PCTs. The research team were not allowed to send the questionnaires directly and had to rely on their distribution via the PCT. This meant a loss of control of the process, and the virtual 'handing over' of the running of the project to the PCT. Since numbers of questionnaires sent could not be provided by the PCT, response rates could not be calculated. Further contact with participants was also made difficult. All these issues led to a devaluing of the quality of the research conducted.

Wray et al. (2006) also experienced similar problems in their study of older nurses. Multi-regional ethical approval was given for the research but the team were denied direct access to contact details of subjects, and thus were obliged to approach the Trusts and PCTs to send out the survey on their behalf, with similar ramifications to those experienced by Leese et al. (2005). Despite receiving ethical approval, some Trusts were unable to send out questionnaires because they were required to participate in the staff survey and felt unable to commit to both. Ethical approval was given in 23 Trusts and PCTs; however, only 13 finally participated. Some were unable to identify staff within the organization that they could distribute the questionnaire to; others did not respond to requests for involvement at all, and two responded after the deadline date and were not able to be included.

Another issue raised by Leese et al. (2005) around the Research Governance process is the rights of the researcher under the Framework. For example, they expressed a belief that it is unethical and against the human rights of the researcher to have personal and health information made available to every PCT in England without assurances of secure storage and appropriate destruction. Also, the Framework infringes on the researcher's 'right to perform their research to the best of their ability' (Leese et al. 2005: 501).

According to the Department of Health:

> the Government is committed to enhancing the contribution of research to health and social care. Research is essential to the successful promotion and protection of health and well-being, and also to modern, effective health and social care services. At the same time, research can involve an element of risk, both in terms of return on investment and sometimes for the safety and well-being of the research participants. Proper governance of research is essential

> to ensure that the public can have confidence in, and benefit from, quality research in health and social care.
>
> (Department of Health 2005: 2)

It appears, however, that this 'proper governance' has been actively impeding high-quality, multi-centre research, hence undermining one of the Framework's main aims. In the current climate, it is quite possible that research on older nurses will be chosen for ease of passage through the governance process, rather than for the quality and content of the research itself. Projects are likely to be small in scale and local, in direct contrast to the intentions and needs of the NHS and the Department of Health. Kielmann et al. (2007: 237) made reference to the 'absurdity of stringent governance requirements', and this will need to be addressed if high-quality, relevant research is to continue to be conducted in the health and social care sector and with their workforces.

Future directions

The ageing of the nursing and midwifery workforce is likely to continue. The concomitant shortage of nurses and midwives is also likely to remain. Given this, more research work needs to be undertaken in this area. The UK also needs to look cross-nationally to learn from the experiences of other countries in Europe, and world-wide. Cross-national research is important in establishing the generality of findings and the validity of interpretations from single-nation studies. Cross-national studies may also reveal patterns and contribute to a further understanding of the phenomenon.

Other phenomena, not considered thus far, will also have a bearing on the nursing workforce in terms of its overall size and these, in turn, are having an effect on the composition of the wider health care workforce. These issues are pertinent in the UK but also across the world. The diminishing nursing workforce is leading governments and health services to question the need for so many registered nurses and, concomitantly, due to pressures on the medical workforce, whether nurses can undertake more specialized and advanced roles. Essentially, the professional nursing workforce is being undermined at both ends of its expertise: at the level of essential caring tasks such as personal care and observation of vital signs by the development of health care assistants and other practitioners (Shields and Watson 2007; Watson 2007), and at the level of quasi-medical tasks by the development of specialist, advanced and nurse consultant roles (Thompson and Watson 2003).

Research needs to be conducted in relation to these phenomena and how they relate to the experience of older nurses. For example, older nurses may view the delegation of essential aspects of care, which were very much the foundation of their own training and nurse education, as abandoning the essential aspects of nursing to people who are not qualified to carry out these tasks. On the other hand, they may question the encroachment of nursing into areas of practice that are traditionally considered to be medical. Advanced roles require considerable continuing professional development and we have already seen how older nurses are disadvantaged in this respect; even if they wanted to undertake advanced roles, there may be a bias towards younger – and less experienced – nurses filling these roles. Whatever the situation regarding the attitude of older nurses towards the changes described above, these changes, which have a significant impact on the professional role of the registered nurse, will compound some of the other difficulties associated with technological and policy-related changes in the NHS that make the return to practice of older nurses difficult.

Bibliography

Ball, J. and Pike, G. (2005) *Managing to Work Differently: Results from the RCN Employment Survey 2005*. London: Royal College of Nursing.

Bardasi, E. and Jenkins, S.P. (2002) *Income in Later Life: Work History Matters*. Bristol: The Policy Press.

Bjork, I.T., Samdal, G.B., Hansen, B.S., Torstad, S. and Hamilton, G.A. (2007) Job satisfaction in a Norwegian population of nurses: a questionnaire survey, *International Journal of Nursing Studies*, 44(5): 747–57.

Buchan, J. (1998) Further flexing? Issues of employment contract flexibility in the UK nursing workforce, *Health Services Management Research*, 11: 148–62.

Buchan, J. (1999) The 'greying' of the United Kingdom nursing workforce: implications for employment policy and practice, *Journal of Advanced Nursing*, 30(4): 818–26.

Buchan, J. (2000) Nursing: a statistical hangover, *Nursing Standard*, 15(13–15): 21–22.

Buchan, J. and Calman, L. (2004) *The Global Shortage of Registered Nurses: An Overview of Issues and Actions*. Geneva: International Council of Nurses (ICN).

Buchan, J. and Seccombe, I. (2005) *Past Trends, Future Imperfect? A Review of the UK Nursing Labour Market 2004/2005*. London: Royal College of Nursing.

Buerhaus, P.I., Staiger, D.O. and Auerbach, D.I. (2000) Implications of an ageing registered nurse workforce, *The Journal of the American Medical Association*, 283(22): 2948–54.

Davies, C. (1995) *Gender and the Professional Predicament in Nursing:* Milton Keynes: Open University Press.

Department of Health (1997) *Non-medical Workforce Census, England: 30 September 1996*. Leeds: NHS Executive.

Department of Health (2000a) *Looking Beyond Labels: Widening the Employment Opportunities for Disabled People in the new NHS*. London: Department of Health.

Department of Health (2000b) *Improving Working Lives Standard*. London: Department of Health.

Department of Health (2001) *Research Governance Framework for Health and Social Care*. London: Department of Health.

Department of Health (2005) *Research Governance Framework for Health and Social Care*, 2nd edn. London: Department of Health.

Elwyn, G., Seagrove, A., Thorne, K. and Cheung, W.Y. (2005) Ethics and research governance in a multicentre study: add 150 days to your study protocol, *British Medical Journal*, 330: 238.

Green, C. (1987) Multiple role women: the real world of the mature RN learner, *Journal of Nursing Education*, 26(7): 266–71.

Hawley, J.M. and Foley, B.J. (2004) Being refreshed: evaluation of a nurse refresher course, *The Journal of Continuing Education in Nursing*, 35(2): 84–88.

Hirsch, D. (2003) *Crossroads After 50: Improving Choices in Work and Retirement*. York: Joseph Rowntree Foundation.

Hirsch, D. (ed.) (2005) *Sustaining Working Lives: A Framework for Policy and Practice*. York: Joseph Rowntree Foundation.

HOPE (2004) Standing Committee of Hospitals of the European Union, *The Healthcare Workforce in Europe: Problems and Solutions*. Brussels: HOPE.

Hornstein, Z., Encel, S., Gunderson, M. and Neumark, D. (2001) *Outlawing Age Discrimination Foreign Lessons, UK Choices*. Bristol: The Policy Press for the Joseph Rowntree Foundation.

House of Lords (2003) *Aspects of the Economics of an Ageing Population*, Vol. 1-Report, HL Paper 179-I, London: HMSO.

Kielmann, T., Tierney, A., Porteous, R., Huby, G., Sheikh, A. and Pinnock, H. (2007) The Department of Health's research governance framework remains an impediment to multi-centre studies: findings from a national descriptive study, *Journal of the Royal Society of Medicine*, 100: 234–38.

Lankshear, A.J., Sheldon, T.A. and Maynard, A. (2005) Nurse staffing and healthcare outcomes: a systematic review of the international research evidence, *Advances in Nursing Science*, 28(2): 163–74.

Leese, B., Storey, C., Ford, J. and Cheater, F. (2005) Researchers' responses to research management and governance for primary care research in England: persistent and escalating problems over time, *Journal of Health Organisation and Management*, 19(6): 494–503.

Lissenburgh, S. and Smeaton, D. (2003) *The Role of Flexible Employment in Maintaining Labour Market Participation and Promoting Job Quality*. York: Joseph Rowntree Foundation.

Loretto, W., Vickerstaff, S. and White, P.J. (2005) *Older Workers and Options for Flexible Work*. Manchester: Equal Opportunities Commission.

Loretto, W., Vickerstaff, S. and White, P. (2006) Introduction themed section: what do older workers want? *Social Policy and Society*, 5(4): 479–83.

Meadows, P. (2002) *Early Retirement and Income in Later Life*. Bristol: The Policy Press for the Joseph Rowntree Foundation.

Mooney, A., Statham, J. and Simon, A. (2002) *The Pivot Generation: Informal Care and Work after 50*. Bristol: The Policy Press for the Joseph Rowntree Foundation.

Newman, K., Maylor, U. and Chansarkar, B. (2001) The nurse retention, quality of care and patient satisfaction chain, *International Journal of Health Care Quality Assurance*, 14(2): 57–68.

OECD (2004) *Towards High Performing Health Systems: Summary Report*. Paris: Organization for Economic Co-operation and Development (OECD).

Pattani, S., Constantinovici, N. and Williams, S. (2001) Who retires early from the NHS because of ill health and what does it cost? A national cross-sectional study, *British Medical Journal*, 322: 208–09.

Phillipson, C. (1998) *Reconstructing Old Age*. London: Sage Publications.

Royal College of Midwives (2006) *Recruitment Shortages in Midwifery 'threatens service'*. Press Release 15 February, London: Royal College of Midwives.

Royal College of Nursing (2001) *Shifting Patterns: A Guide to Employee-friendly Working*. London: Royal College of Nursing.

Royal College of Nursing (2003) *More Nurses, Working Differently? A Review of the UK Nursing Labour Market 2002–2003*. London: Royal College of Nursing.

Salisbury, C., Leese, B. and McManus, R.J. (2005) Ensuring that research governance supports rather than stifles research, *British Journal of General Practice*, 55: 4–5.

Sandall, J. (1998) Occupational burnout in midwives: new ways of working and the relationship between organizational factors and psychological health and well-being, *Risk Decision and Policy*, 3(3): 213–32.

Shields, L. and Watson, R. (2007) The demise of nursing in the United Kingdom: a warning for medicine, *Journal of the Royal Society of Medicine*, 100: 70–74.

Storey, H.C., Ford, J., Cheater, F., Harding, N., Buchan, J., Hurst, K. and Leese, B. (2007) *Improving the Retention of Women in the Primary and Community Care Nursing Workforce After the Age of Fifty Years*. NHS Employers (www.nhsemployers.org/excellence/excellence-482.cfm).

Taylor, P. (2002) *New Policies for Older Workers*. Bristol: The Policy Press for the Joseph Rowntree Foundation.

Thompson, D.R. and Watson, R. (2003) Advanced nursing practice: what is it? *International Journal of Nursing Practice*, 9: 129–30.

Vickerstaff, S., Baldock, J., Cox, J. and Keen, L. (2004) *Happy Retirement? The Impact of Employers' Policies and Practice on the Process of Retirement*. Bristol: The Policy Press for the Joseph Rowntree Foundation.

Victor, C.R. and Khakoo, A.A. (1994) Is hospital the right place? A survey of 'inappropriate' admissions to an inner London NHS Trust, *Journal of Public Health Medicine*, 16(3): 286–90.

Watson, R. (2007) Do HCAs deskill nurses? YES, *British Journal of Healthcare Assistants*, 1: 58.

Watson, R., Manthorpe, J. and Andrews, J. (2003) *Nurses Over 50: Options, Decisions and Outcomes*. Bristol: The Policy Press for the Joseph Rowntree Foundation.

WHO (2004) High Level Forum on the Health MDGs, *Summary of Discussions and Agreed Action Points*, Geneva: World Health Organization (WHO) High Level Forum.

Wray, J., Watson, R., Stimpson, A., Gibson, H. and Aspland, J. (2006) *'A Wealth of Knowledge': The Employment Experiences of Older Nurses, Midwives and the NHS*. Hull: The University of Hull.

Index

WOMEN IN LATER LIFE

Exploring Race and Ethnicity

Mary Maynard, Haleh Afshar, Myfanwy Franks and Sharon Wray

'... the first book to comprehensively examine the lives of older women from ethnic minorities in the UK as well as non-migrant White women. The authors draw on extensive qualitative research to provide novel ways of looking at the priorities and concerns of older women, providing insights into what enhances their quality of life. Mary Maynard and colleagues have written an outstanding book ... Women in Later Life will be essential reading for students on undergraduate and postgraduate courses on gender, ethnicity and later life.'

Sara Arber, University of Surrey

'... what is it like to be an older person and, particularly, an older woman? This carefully crafted and wide-ranging book seeks to answer this question ...The book reminds us that age is a social construct, one which profoundly disadvantages women. For minority ethnic women, where this book makes an important contribution to a largely unexplored territory, the situation is even more dire. The authors have opened up a huge area of policy, demonstrating, despite the rhetoric of government, how badly we treat our elders.'

Professor Gary Craig, University of Hull

Britain, along with other Western and industrialized countries, has an ageing population. We already live in one of the demographically oldest societies to have ever existed and the population is going to get older. By 2020 it is estimated that one third of the population will be aged over 50. Furthermore, older women outnumber older men, since men tend to die at a younger age than women.

In the academic mainstream relatively little is known about older women from minority ethnic communities. This groundbreaking book is based on interviews and focus groups with women of different backgrounds and ethnicities whose lives illustrate the strength of character and optimism that have often enabled them to live through hard times but who, in general, view later life positively.

In seeking to understand the relationships between age, gender and ethnicity, the authors focus on a number of key themes including:

- Family and networks
- Health and well being
- Religion, faith and spirituality
- Income, pensions and housing
- The meaning of identity and life course events
- Death and dying

Women in Later Life will be key reading for students and practitioners with an interest in gender and/or issues surrounding later life.

Contents: *Introduction – The lives of older women – Studying older women: Issues of theory and methodology – Identities and life course events – Family networks and the moral economy of kin – Health and well-being – Faith and identity – Death, dying and widowhood – Concluding remarks.*

2008 208pp

978-0-335-21525-6 (Paperback) 978-0-335-21526-3 (Hardback)

THE SOCIAL WORLD OF OLDER PEOPLE

Understanding Loneliness and Social Isolation in Later Life

Christina Victor, Sasha Scambler and John Bond

Developments to the physical environment, scientific and technological innovation, the reorganisation of work and leisure and the impact of globalization and global capitalism have all influenced the nature of the world in which we now live. Social engagement and relationships, however, remain important at any age and their quality is a key element contributing to the quality of life of older people.

This book provides a detailed account of loneliness and social isolation as experienced by older people living in Britain. The authors consider the incidence and effects of isolation and loneliness, identifying the factors which lead to such experiences and considering potential interventions. They also argue that these feelings are experienced at all stages of the life course and not unique to the social world of older people.

Victor, Scambler and Bond rationalise that this is an important area, as both loneliness and social isolation are negatively associated with both quality and quantity of life – whilst the maintenance of social relationships is seen as a key component of 'successful ageing'.

The Social World of Older People is important reading for students of social work, gerontology, community care and social policy as well as being of interest to policy makers and practitioners in these fields.

Contents: *Preface and Acknowledgements - Introduction - Loneliness and social isolation: Issues of theory and method - Social relations and everyday life - Experiences of loneliness - Social exclusion and social isolation - Rethinking loneliness and social isolation in later life – References – Index.*

2008 232pp

978-0-335-21521-8 (Paperback) 978-0-335-21522-5 (Hardback)

GROWING OLDER IN EUROPE

Alan Walker (ed)

This book provides a comprehensive picture of quality of life in old age in five very different European Union countries. Based on systematic review of the evidence in Germany, Italy, the Netherlands, Sweden and the UIKL by leading national experts the volume constitutes a unique resource for anyone interested in ageing in Europe.

As well as covering all the most important issues concerning quality in later life, including physical and mental health, the environments of ageing, employment and income, family and support networks and participation and social integration, each chapter follows a standard format to ensure maximum accessibility of the material presented and comparisons between the countries. A comparative framework is provided in the introductory chapter which also places the five countries in their broad European context.

The research evidence contained in this volume has never been available previously in the one place and, therefore, it represents a unique contribution to the literature. The book is intended as a companion volume to the others in the *Growing Older* series providing the only comparative European perspective.

This comparative analysis shows that many similar quality of later life issues are being faced by older people in different EU countries but that the policy and service contexts are quite different, as are the research traditions.

Contents: List of contributors – Preface – Part 1. Quality of life in old age in Europe – Quality of life in old age: Definitions, environments and socio-economic aspects – Germany: Quality of life in old age – Italy: Quality of life in old age – The Netherlands: Quality of life in old age – Sweden: Quality of life in old age – UK: Quality of life in old age – Part II: Quality of life in old age: Participation, social support and subjective well-being – Germany: Quality of life in old age – Italy: Quality of life in old age – The Netherlands: Quality of life in old age – Sweden: Quality of life in old age – UK: Quality of life in old age – References – Index.

2004 312pp

978-0-335-21513-3 (Paperback) 978-0-335-21514-0 (Hardback)